In Search of T

A Portrait of Don C

E B Adams

Royal Society of Medicine Services Limited

Royal Society of Medicine Services Limited
1 Wimpole Street London W1M 8AE
8 East 60th Street New York NY 10022

British Library Cataloguing in Publication Data

Adams, E. B.
In search of truth: a portrait of Don Craib.
1. South Africa. Medicine. Craib, Don 1896-1982
I. Title
610′.92′4

ISBN 1-85315-119-X
ISBN 1-85315-118-1 (pbk)

Library of Congress Cataloging-in-Publication Data

Adams, E. B. (E. Barry), 1918–
In search of truth.

1. Craib, Hofmeyr William, 1896–1982. 2. Physicians –South Africa–Biography. I. Title.
R654.C73A35 1989 610.92 [B] 89-70140
ISBN 1-85315-119-X
ISBN 1-85315-118-1 (pbk)

Editorial and production services by Diane Crofter-Harris, Devizes, Wiltshire

Phototypeset by Dobbie Typesetting Limited, Plymouth, Devon

Printed in Great Britain by Henry Ling Ltd, at the Dorset Press, Dorchester

Contents

List of Illustrations

Acknowledgements

Mrs Doris Craib generously gave me access to all her husband's letters, unpublished memoirs and the numerous other documents which form the basis of this book. I thank her for this and for much other assistance she has given me in my task, happily undertaken.

I am also indebted to many others who have helped me, especially my wife for her patience and constructive criticism; Mary Davidson, Don Craib's niece, and her husband Dr Fred Davidson, who discussed this fascinating man with me on many occasions during the writing; and Tom Bothwell, who really initiated the project and always supported my efforts.

Apart from those already mentioned, permission to quote from their letters to Don Craib over the years (which he had meticulously kept), or from memoranda or papers they had written relating to Craib in some way was freely given by the following, whom I thank: Dr Raymond Pruitt; Professor Bruce Murray; Professor James Gear; Dr John Honour; Dr Christopher Lewis; Dr Howard Burchell; Mrs Patsy Skinner; Mr Murray Baxter; Johns Hopkins University Press; British Heart Journal; Royal College of Physicians, London; Mrs EA Shepherd.

Photographs for inclusion in this book were kindly made available by Mrs Doris Craib; Dr Mary Davidson; Dr Arthur Hollman; Mr Sinclair Watson; Lord Adrian; Miss Elizabeth Hunkin; Professor TH Bothwell; University of the Witwatersrand; the South African Medical Research Council; Mrs P Skinner.

For their considerable assistance I also wish to thank Sir Christopher Booth, President of the Royal Society of Medicine; and Mr Brian Weight and Mrs Diane Crofter-Harris, of Royal Society of Medicine Services Limited, who have seen this slim volume into print.

E B Adams
October 1989

To my friend Tom Bothwell
and my wife Sybil

Preface

The fabric of this book is woven around the life of a man of outstanding gifts. Not the least of these were the clarity of his mind and the warmth of his personality. Of Scottish Craib and Afrikaner Hofmeyr parentage, he was born in the small Karoo town of Somerset East in Cape colonial days, and died there 86 years later (in 1982). Despite his given names, William Hofmeyr, all his life he was affectionately known as Don or Donal. Clear of mind though infirm of body, when death came he was greatly revered at home and abroad for his contributions to medicine, and much loved by a wide circle of family and friends. He was delightful to meet for his friendship, his wit and his scintillating conversation; but judged from letters and much unpublished material he left behind, until the end he relived and was disturbed by some of the controversy which surrounded his scientific career. But he was a man of many parts and his story is worth telling.

In outline, his formative years were spent on a farm near Somerset East where he was surrounded by a close-knit family of considerable ability. Many members of his mother's family— Hofmeyrs and Murrays—had made great contributions to South African history. A Presbyterian minister, Andrew Murray had come from Scotland to help the Dutch Reformed Church and became a distinguished religious leader; the young Craib's grandfather ministered to the

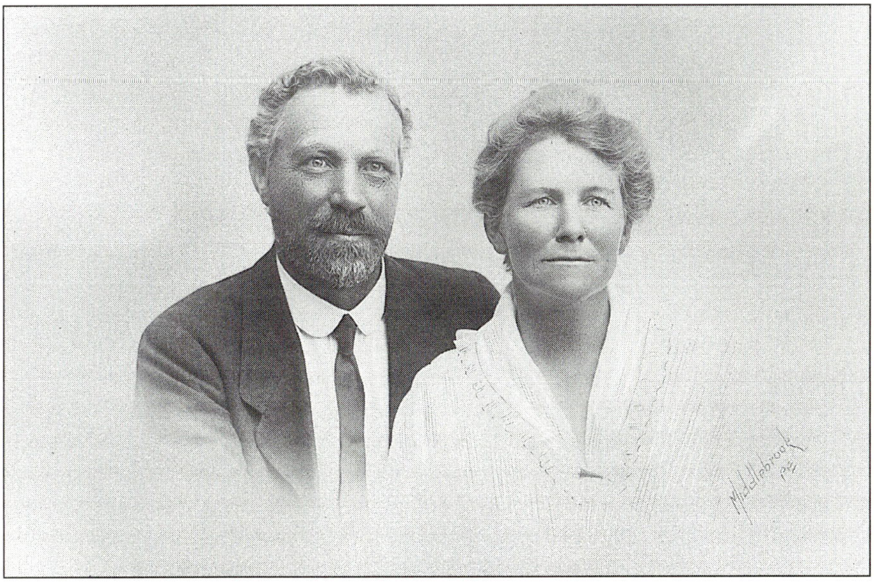

Don's parents, James and Isabella Craib.

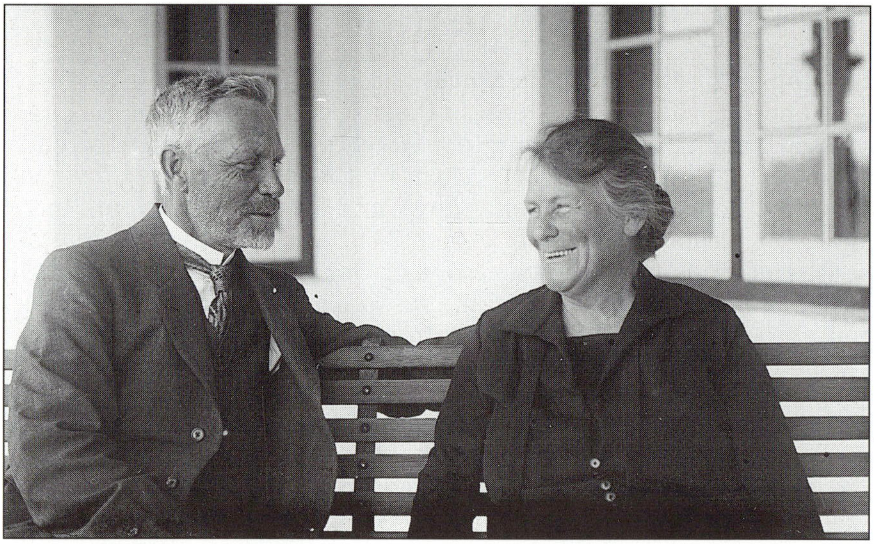

Don's parents in jocular mood.

people of Somerset East for many years; and several of his uncles were also dominees. Although baptised in his Hofmeyr grandfather's church, Don grew up a Presbyterian, the denomination to which his father, James Craib, belonged. Don's religious upbringing was undoubtedly Calvinistic, and his first great intellectual challenge, as will be seen, arose in his childhood out of what he was told of the Crucifixion. His mother, Isabella, was a remarkable woman, erudite and wise; and she and her eldest son, Don, spent long hours in conversation.

Like Andrew Murray, Don's father had come from Scotland to the Cape; not to help the church but to teach at Gill College in Somerset East, in the days when several schools in South Africa offered university courses towards a degree at the University of the Cape of Good Hope. Schooled at Gill, Don early showed his intellectual calibre by coming first in the Cape matriculation examination in 1911 and, in 1914, gaining honours when he graduated BA at the South African College (now the University of Cape Town). His majors were mathematics, applied mathematics and physics; his original intention was to become an engineer. In the First World War he was in South West Africa with the South African forces, and in France with the British Army. Here he distinguished himself as a trench mortar officer, being twice mentioned in despatches and awarded the Military Cross and Bar. A seasoned soldier and intellectually mature, he went up to Cambridge when peace came, later qualifying in medicine from Guy's Hospital, London.

By the time he was a registrar in the medical wards at Guy's, he had clearly impressed the consultant staff; and it is probable that nobody was surprised when he was awarded a coveted Rockefeller

Fellowship to Johns Hopkins Hospital, Baltimore. Here he carried out his now-famous experiments on isolated animal heart muscle. From these he formulated his doublet hypothesis. Though brilliant in its simplicity and logic, his work brought him into confrontation with acknowledged leaders in the field. After Baltimore, he went back to London, continuing his researches in electrophysiology under Sir Thomas Lewis. His incisive thinking and unassailable logic led to clashes with authority, in particular with Einthoven, the great Dutch researcher who was doyen of all European workers in electrocardiology; Lord Adrian, Professor of Physiology at Cambridge; and even Lewis, whom he greatly admired.

His doublet hypothesis apparently rejected, and feeling himself personally discredited and regarded as a fraud, he turned down several attractive offers of academic or research posts away from Lewis's laboratories at University College Hospital, determined to return to South Africa and abandon his ambition to spend his life in electrophysiological research. So 1931 saw him back home in Somerset East, newly married to Doris Vevers, a young woman of great charm and a 'cellist of considerable ability whom he had met in London and who was to share the rest of his life with him.

Heralded by bitter controversy for which he cannot be held responsible, his appointment to the chair of medicine at the University of the Witwatersrand proved a conspicuous success. To this scores of his medical students in Johannesburg and hundreds of medical men in various parts of the world would readily testify; and with gratitude, for he taught them a philosophy of thinking about medical problems and challenging currently held theories which profoundly influenced their professional lives. Moreover, he is remembered with affection, for he was a striking personality with a great zest for life and an endearing sense of humour. Some of the anecdotes attributed to him became a legend in his time at Wits* and afterwards when he had moved on. Several are related elsewhere in this book.

As in his years in medical research at Johns Hopkins in Baltimore and in Lewis's clinical research laboratories in London, controversy again surrounded him in his fifteen years as Professor of Medicine (1932–1947). Appointed on a part-time basis, he vigorously pressed for the establishment of full-time clinical departments. He wanted to lift them from what he regarded as provincial mediocrity to a level where their teaching and research would match that of the best abroad. But he was again well ahead of his time and was frequently frustrated in his attempts to mould the medical school to fit his visionary plans. Nevertheless, with minimal staff to assist him and no research facilities, he stimulated students and his younger colleagues by his penetrating questions and his lucid thinking at

*Wits is the commonly used colloquial name for the University of the Witwatersrand.

the bedside, establishing himself as a dominant figure in South African clinical medicine.

Ironically, when clinical full-time staff establishments were finally created in 1946, Craib did not put his name forward as he felt, with some justification, that many in authority in the university were opposed to him. Before the Second World War he had been obliged for financial reasons to share his academic work with practice as a consultant physician in Johannesburg, but during the war he had served as a part-time colonel in the South African Medical Corps. Feeling that he had been squeezed out of Wits, he had no heart for returning to private practice in Johannesburg. Instead, he went to Port Elizabeth where he practised for many years. His new milieu had the advantage for him that it was not far from Gardiol, the family farm outside Somerset East, his birthplace.

His expertise as a research worker and his clear analytical mind had not been forgotten, however, for the Council for Scientific and Industrial Research eventually invited him to become one of its Vice-Presidents, charging him with the promotion of medical research in South Africa. Based in Pretoria, he performed this task with distinction and conspicuous success. When he retired at the age of seventy-three he had spent, he said, some of his happiest and most fulfilling years in this research environment.

An attractive little place, Somerset East nestles below one of the many mountains scattered across the Little Karoo. It might be described as part of the platteland of South Africa, the outback. Somewhat dominated by its handsome Dutch Reformed Church of traditional design, with a main street and many of the homesteads distinctly Victorian in architecture, the town combines quiet charm with an air of living in the past. Its people appear to be warm and friendly and it is probably true to say that in general their outlook would be distinctly conservative. Here Don Craib chose to live out his life, happy to be back again on Gardiol, his farm a few miles out of town. In the event some thirteen years remained for him, and physical infirmities forced the Craibs to sell their home of so many years and move into a house in town two years before he died.

Don Craib clearly loved the physical environment of Somerset East but he felt intellectually isolated, a disadvantage he attempted to rectify by copious letter-writing. He corresponded with hundreds of former students and colleagues in South Africa and abroad; with philosophers and lawyers and religious leaders; and with many others. What he wrote about was usually topical. Quite often, however, it concerned his intellectually turbulent past and the controversies which had surrounded him. He usually wrote without rancour and often in an apparently jocular way; but his letters were fundamentally deep and searching. Frequently he would question the precise meaning of terms and ask others for their opinions.

Running through most of his correspondence, in substance or implied, was Craib in search of truth.

He taught me medicine at the University of the Witwatersrand and I fell under his spell. He profoundly influenced my thinking, which is perhaps the ultimate goal of any teacher. He became my friend later on, and a year before his death my wife and I travelled to see him at his home. It was our express purpose to record on tape something of his past struggles and the thoughts so often reflected in his letters. This was a pleasant task undertaken for the archives at Wits at the suggestion of Professor TH Bothwell—and with his active support. Like Don Craib before him, Tom Bothwell holds the chair of medicine in the university, which he has served with distinction and gained international recognition for his researches in iron metabolism. The tapes and a transcription in book form (*Discussions with William Hofmeyr Craib*) have been lodged in the medical library in Johannesburg, and there are copies of the transcription in the archives of the university and in the Adler Museum of the History of Medicine.

After Don's death we went back to Somerset East to stay in his wife's charming home; this time to help sort out his voluminous papers and correspondence. We found that he had kept copies of countless personal letters written over the span of many years, as well as a large number of letters he had received. In his study there were also numerous manuscripts and fragments he had composed about his life and the people with whom he had come in contact. Perhaps he had had in mind a book of memoirs. Several times, he had said, others had asked his permission to write his biography, which he had refused. The fragments found in memoir form in his study after his death were never published.

This pen picture attempts to portray Don Craib the man. It is not a biography, for including the more conventional details of a full biography would have detracted from the aims the author had in mind when he set out on his task. The goal was to depict this fascinating, deeply-thinking yet fun-loving man for others to enjoy and perhaps be intrigued by; and at the same time to relate him to the times in which he lived. He did not appear to be against such a book when we recorded what he had to say about his life at Somerset East in 1982. Wherever possible, his story is told in his own words in the pages that follow.

Chapter 1

Gardiol

Don Craib grew up at Gardiol, the family farm a few miles outside Somerset East. The homestead still stands, only vacated by the Craibs in recent years when old age dictated the wisdom of living in the town. Indeed, Gardiol was to be Don's home, off and on, throughout his life; when not his actual place of residence, at least the sanctum to which he returned to keep alive the family ties which obviously meant so much to him.

Somerset East is in the Karoo, a gently rolling plateau towards the southern tip of Africa. Here and there lie scattered mountain ranges of great beauty. Although semi-arid, it is full of fascinating plant and insect life, and once teemed with large herds of wild animals. It is excellent for sheep farming. The town's ambience must have been similar in the closing years of the nineteenth century, for its old homes and some of its public buildings are clearly Victorian; and it has not grown much. In South Africa it would rank as a dorp, a widely-used Afrikaans word for a country town or village. In her *Dictionary of South African English*, Jean Branford adds that it is sometimes used in a derogatory sense to mean a backward or unprogressive place. Some big city dwellers would certainly regard Somerset East as such, but the author was impressed by its grace and its quiet dignity during visits there in the 1970s and 1980s. He was also struck by the physical dominance of the imposing Dutch Reformed Church, a statue of a Hofmeyr (Don's grandfather) commanding its entrance; and by the realisation that Somerset East is just as much a part of the fabric of South African history as the Castle in Cape Town, the battlefield at Isandhlwana, or the mines in Johannesburg.

James Craib, teaching at Gill College in Somerset East, must have married one of his former students, for it was here that Isabella Cornelia Hofmeyr obtained a Bachelor of Arts degree in 1893: a pioneer woman graduate in South Africa. She studied at night by candlelight at her father's home, 'Die Pastorie'; chewing dried apricots, she would later recall, to keep her awake. Don was their first child. During his youth they bought a small farm outside the town and planted many oak trees there, naming their new home Gardiol. The name comes from Jean Jacques Gardiol, one of the Huguenots who fled to the Cape from religious persecution in France. It is said that he brought acorns with him, planting them on the tract of land granted him by the Governor, Simon van der Stel, determined to make his farm beautiful. One of the oaks he planted

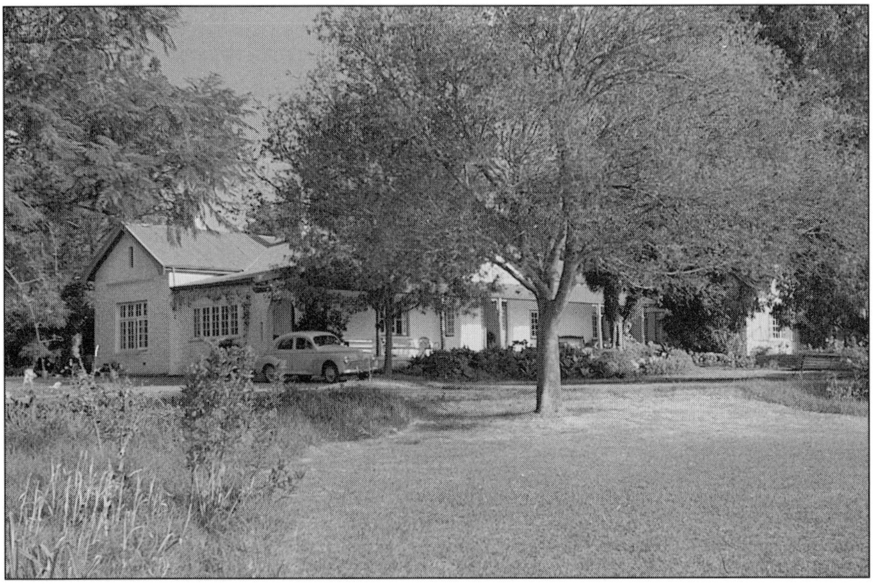

Gardiol, Somerset East.

in 1694 still stands. The Craibs intended to beautify their home by similar means.

It is difficult to paint a picture of Craib's boyhood after all these years without access to contemporaries or better documentation, but some help about the Craib family home has come from recollections kindly given to the author by Mary Davidson. 'Our family always went to Gardiol, my grandmother's farm,' she wrote, referring to the 1930s and 1940s, 'for the long December and mid-year holidays, and Don Craib, my uncle, and his family were usually there at Christmas, and sometimes at other times as well. The farm was situated three miles south of Somerset East, and the Little Fish River skirted its boundary in a wide loop. The name of the farm was derived from Jean Jacques Gardiol who came to South Africa with the Huguenots. During the Second World War my parents were away in Britain, and I and my sister and brother were looked after by my grandmother, and the farm was our home. After the war, Don took over the running of the farm and visited there more and more often, until it became his home when my grandmother died in 1967.

'My grandmother was the central figure in the family for over half a century. We called her Ouma; she had been christened Cornelia Isabella but her sisters called her Isie. She had five children, of whom Don was the eldest. Oupa, her husband, died in 1938.

'Gardiol was the centre of many family gatherings, usually at Christmas-time. We often sat down to meals twelve or fifteen in number; in addition, small children were fed on the verandah or in the kitchen. Ouma must have been hard-pressed at times to accommodate everyone, and three rondavels were built behind the main house as extra bedrooms. After the war, Don added on a new wing of beautiful design which provided about five extra rooms.

'During the day, tennis, swimming and walks were the main occupations. Bridge and chess and a type of word-game were played in the evenings. Now and then a mountain climb in the nearby Boschberg or a picnic in the kloof at Bester's Hoek was arranged. As the custom was to have large hot midday meals, it was expected of everyone that they rest from about two until half-past four. As the summer day cooled down, people emerged from their bedrooms for tea or tennis, or an inspection of the farm. Don and his sisters and brothers inherited the Hofmeyr love of gardening, and progress in the flower and vegetable gardens was followed with keen interest. The wonderful flavour of these holiday times was given by the combination of sporting pursuits, large wonderful meals and long discussions between Ouma and her children.

'Conversation in the family never flagged. My uncles and my parents were often in deep discussion and conducted long debates with each other. Don and Murray were doctors, Ian a forestry expert, my father a physicist and my mother an historian. We all thought that Ouma was the wisest person of all. She and her children, particularly Don, strolled in the garden deep in conversation—after breakfast or in the late afternoons. Don and Ouma often had quiet discussions in the evenings after Ouma had gone to bed. Don used to sit beside her bed, and in the bedroom next door I would hear the murmur of their voices, and every now and then Don's laugh, as I went to sleep.'

Mary Davidson's recollections of Gardiol, and of her discussions with Don, often disagreeing with him, have their influence elsewhere in this book, but perhaps it is worth recording now a vivid memory she has about her eldest Craib uncle. 'I always felt', she wrote, 'that Don's intelligent face, neat features, level eyes and tanned skin made him most handsome. His perceptiveness and humour gave him compelling personal charisma, which even today has never faded. The special thing about him was his passion for exchanging ideas.'

It was in his childhood at Gardiol that Craib began to challenge the things about him with a clarity of mind which became his most outstanding attribute. He was brought up, he recalled, 'in a very, very Calvinistic atmosphere; very much in an intense odour of sanctity . . . My grandfather was a minister in the Dutch Reformed Church, to which I was initially taken.' At an early age he was apparently told in a dogmatic way that the Jews had crucified Christ; and he took this to be implied in the literal sense. 'I discovered at the time I was about ten and able to read the *Bible* for myself that I had been told something that was not true. The Roman soldiers were the ones who crucified Jesus, while we in Somerset East were

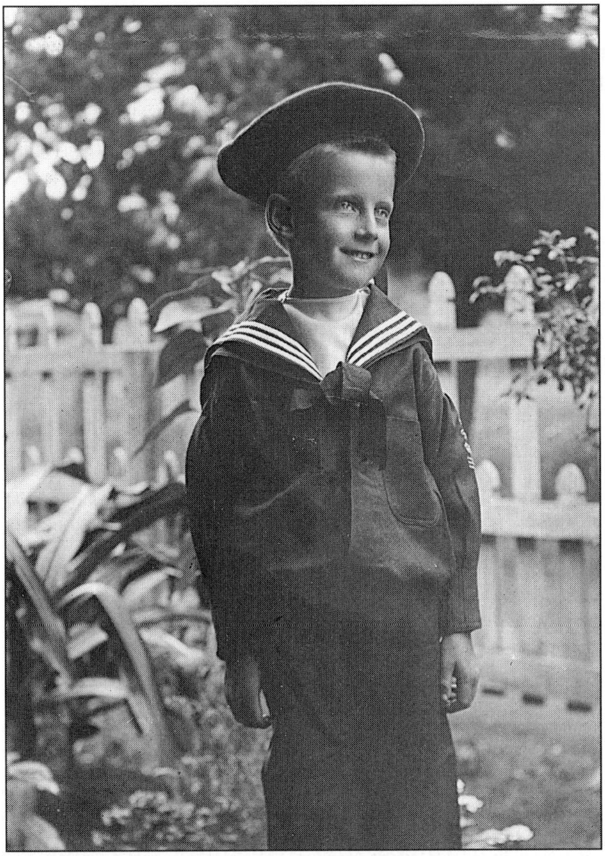

Don Craib the boy. Not long after this he started challenging the teaching of his elders.

being brought up to believe that the Jews were the . . . frightful people who crucified Jesus. It shook me a bit when I first tumbled to this fact, for I then began to observe that all my adult mentors, all my adult teachers, were lying to me on this particular point.

'Having decided that adults were lying to me, I began to listen to them as they talked and I found that it was true in a number of other instances I could easily name now, that they were telling me something that was not true, did not fit in with historical fact as I understood "historical fact" to mean. For example, I was informed that the *Bible* was the infallible word of God—not a single word in it did not come direct from God to man—that is how we were brought up to understand it. Then having found this one error, I said to myself that if I call all these people liars, including my mother and father and all the rest of them, what is the meaning of the word "truth"?

'I began to be very worried about truth; and I left school with a fixed idea in my mind that truth is in no way different from fact, reality, event. As soon as a person made a statement that did not agree with or was not consistent with fact, reality, event, it was not truth. And I found by the time I matriculated that there was never argument when there was discussion of fact, reality, event. Argument always started when opinions were expressed, when hypotheses were put forward, explanations given, guesses made, etc, etc. . . .

'I formed a fixed idea at the time that truth is self-evident. Truth does not depend upon the mind of man for its establishment or for its abolition. You cannot produce truth with words. Truth is independent of man's brain. I left school with this fixed in my mind and I said I will never again tell a lie—I will stick to the facts, realities, events as closely as I can. And to tell the truth to me then meant, not an opinion, not an authoritative statement, but something in keeping with the environment around me.'

These, of course, are memories of Craib's thinking processes recalled seventy years later. It may well be that he had not formulated them so clearly in his youth. Nevertheless, they may be described as the credo upon which much of his subsequent intellectual life was based, as will be seen.

His criticism of the religious dogma of his elders during his boyhood should, however, be seen in perspective. Many of his letters from Britain and the United States in the 1920s revealed deep feelings of attachment to his home and great warmth towards his parents and his brothers and sisters. And at least some of his passion for discussion of all manner of topics throughout his life must have come from the many discussions at Gardiol, as recalled by Mary Davidson.

We visited Gardiol in 1974. Mature oaks lined the drive and a huge Holm oak and many other trees were scattered round the house. In asking us to come for 'a day, a week, a month or a year', Don had written that we should bring Shakespeare and a Tolstoy with us because they had few books in the house, living quietly as they did in the country: a rather typical piece of Craibian humour! In the event we found books everywhere. There was quiet elegance in the lounge and an adjoining sun room, and hundreds if not thousands of volumes lined the walls. There was a small grand piano on which stood pictures of Doris with her 'cello, and some of Don's own paintings hung on the walls. The generously wide verandahs were a conspicuous feature of the house; and it was here before breakfast that Don joined his guests to continue a conversation started at dinner the evening before. He brought with him notes jotted down at midnight on an envelope. These revealed deep understanding of the personality we were discussing, and he put forward a penetrating analysis of the human problems involved. He did not sit in judgement about others as a rule but tried to present the facts as he understood them, interpreting them, as was his habit, in what was almost a separate exercise. One of us had recently been ill and he showed genuine concern—and provided the correct diagnosis of an unusual, distressing, but fortunately benign condition while its history, at his insistence, was being told. Unlike many old people, he invariably kept the conversation away from himself and displayed deep interest in the wellbeing of others.

It was only in his writings that introspection came through.

Chapter 2

Craib at War

Don Craib was caught up in both world wars and his experiences throw a fascinating light on his character and on the times in which he lived. In his later years he set pen to paper on many facets of his life, writing frankly and without ambiguity. He must seriously have considered writing an autobiography, but perhaps because of modesty about his own attainments and consideration for the feelings of those whose paths he crossed, this task was never completed. He certainly held forthright views about others (sometimes expressed in conversation or written in personal memoranda and letters) but at the same time he displayed an old-world courtesy towards them. This appears to be one of the reasons why almost all of what he wrote remained unpublished, for Don would not have wanted to soften or omit what he perceived as the truth for the sake of publication.

After his death I found among his papers several memoranda about his involvement in both world wars. Much of this can be quoted without editing.

World War 1: South-West Africa

Seeking a career in engineering, Craib left Somerset East in 1912 for the South African College (now the University of Cape Town). He had apparently chosen civil engineering so that he could 'dam the flood waters of the usually dry river beds of the Karoo for purposes of conservation and irrigation'. But this was not to be. Events in Europe, 7000 miles away, began 'to play havoc with our young lives' half way through what was to be his final year. For his first two and a half years at university, he wrote, 'the content of such political discussions as took place among undergraduates generally, strange as it now may seem, had little to do with inter-racial strife between the divergent races of our mother country, British, Boer, Asiatic, Coloured, Chinese, Bantu and Indian. Political debate centred largely on the Yellow Peril by which we meant the threat to South Africa, Africa and Australia from the Chinese and Japanese peoples to the East.' He believed that it was during World War 1 that his generation first began to think and to talk about the future relationship between Boer and British in South Africa, and to have profound misgivings as to the wisdom or otherwise of applying the British one man one vote form of democracy to a 'non-homogeneous mixture of races, civilised, semi-civilised and completely primitive'.

The outbreak of war in August 1914 found him half way through a course for the BA degree in Cape Town, majoring in mathematics, physics and applied mathematics, while at the same time apparently taking some engineering subjects. He was called up for active service. Stationed with the Cape Peninsula Rifles near Simonstown, he became company cook: an occupation not likely to satisfy so adventurous a spirit. After temporary leave to enable him to sit the final examinations, he volunteered for active service beyond the country's borders.

Craib was posted to Walvis Bay, with a close friend, JP de Villiers. Both were given the rank of sergeant with equipment for testing sources of water likely to be poisoned by the retreating Germans during the South African advance into South West Africa.

'Unfortunately, on arrival at the front,' he wrote, 'JP and I found that base headquarters at the Cape had in error sent two sergeant analysts when only one such post remained unfilled. As JP had majored in chemistry, while I was a mere mathematician and physicist, I naturally withdrew in commendable dignity, adding that I would like to be returned to the ranks as a private and posted to any regiment going into action, whether infantry, cavalry, artillery, mounted or unmounted, wherever there was an opening for a recruit. "Your only choice", I was informed, "lies between coastal defence at the Cape in your present rank, or active service in the sanitary corps now being formed, with the rank of corporal. Your duties will consist of taking command of a platoon or company of sanitary orderlies consisting of redundant details from various Non-European regiments, now being collected and organised for the purpose. Your duties will involve care and proper sanitary management of the bucket system convenience of the headquarters staff and of such other latrines as are allotted to you." Needless to say this was a heaven sent opportunity to avoid an ignominious return to the Cape, and equally needless to say, Swakopmund soon smelt like a rose!

'In due course the campaign under the command of General Botha got under way and the spearhead of the advance notified of zero hour. Two days prior to the order to move, I had, to my surprise, been relieved of latrine supervision and promoted to become batman and general factotum to Major DG Maynard, SAMC, Deputy Assistant Director of the Medical Services, provided with a horse and saddle, and included in the lower ranks of the headquarters personnel. In due course we were off, travelling by night and resting by day, on the heels of the Germans, who, fighting a rearguard action, slowly withdrew inland and to the north.

'Having no weapon and taking part in no battle, my adventures and experiences in the South-West Africa campaign are of little interest to anyone but myself. Suffice it to say I fulfilled my duties as batman to Major Maynard until after the surrender of the German forces to General Botha just south of the Etosha pan, but was soon afterwards rejected by him as unserviceable, and in disgrace, during the early days of the long trek back from Otavifontein in the north to the base harbour at Walvis Bay in the south.

'The way of it is a story that does me no credit. Not wishing to return to the coast at snail's pace for hundreds of miles in a dust-drenched column many miles long, Major Maynard decided to travel cross-country. A Captain Potter, myself and a native driver in charge of a suitably-laden scotchcart drawn by four mules, as well as three riding horses for ourselves, were detailed to accompany him. The Major intended to use only a compass and military map as guides. The roads shown on the map turned out at times to be nothing but indistinct tracks. As we always travelled at night to avoid the heat of the day, often over wide stretches of barren veld, it was not surprising that one dark night early on in our cross-country odyssey, the Major had to admit that we were lost. He and Captain Potter then went into conference, while the driver and I discussed what we thought was the right thing to do. The Major's orders were in due course delivered. These seemed so strange to the ears of a young colonial, born and bred in the veld, hardly as yet civilised by his few years at Cape Town, that he thought it only right, with all due respect, to point out a more practical procedure to his commanding officer. He quietly suggested that if it was the intention of the Major that a certain mountain range some ten to twelve miles away had to be crossed, it might be a good plan to take a certain course. The Major was not pleased, and summarily ordered his batman to carry out the orders he had already given. The batman thereupon mounted his horse, saluted in style and disappeared into the night. He knew that whatever course the Major, Captain Potter and the driver felt called upon to take, they had eventually to cross the range ahead at its lowest point. In due course the batman reached the road as it passed over the gap, a gap that had been barely visible against the starlit sky from many miles away. There he dismounted, lit his pipe, climbed a highish rock at the roadside and waited.

'An hour or so later the rest of the party arrived. The Major met me with a shattering blast to the effect that he could have me shot at dawn for disobedience to a superior officer while on active service and asked what I had to say for myself. My reply I am afraid did nothing to mollify him and he gave me a further piece of his mind in magnificent, fiery Oxford English, ending with the words: "As punishment you shall walk by the side of your horse for the rest of the night." Not unmoved by the technical justice of his condemnation, but definitely irritated by the heat thereof, I remained silent for a while and then burst out. "Sir," I said, "my advice was sound, as both you and I have proved by meeting here on the road we had lost. I admit the justice of your anger, but dislike the tone of your remarks. You are merely taking advantage of your rank in venting your spleen (how proud I was of these words) upon me, a mere batman. But I tell you now, I'll henceforth carry out to the letter every reasonable order you give me; I'll faithfully do everything I have to do for you as your batman; but not again will I address one single word to you for the rest of our journey to the coast."

'And that's how it was. Such is the arrogance of a Scot, founded on vanity and pride, said by some to be man's greatest sin. For many days and nights I prepared his bed, his food and his bathwater, washed his socks and underwear, looked after him when ill with dysentery, but I never spoke to him again. On arrival at Swakopmund on the coast I was dismissed as a batman and thrown ignominiously into a camp of unwanted and uncared-for base details who had fallen by the wayside or been unable for one reason or another to stand up to the rigours of the campaign. We eventually reached Cape Town, covered in lice and filth accumulated in the overcrowded hold of a German transport, set aside for the voyage south, and were forthwith given temporary leave.

'Major Maynard generously brought no charge against me. He was, moreover, kind enough not long afterwards to give me a written testimonial to accompany my application for acceptance as an officer in a regiment of London Territorials that was then being organised in Britain for active service in France.

'I reached London towards the end of 1915, having paid my passage with £ 100 borrowed on a life insurance policy for £ 500, taken out by my father and handed in as security . . . I had hardly arrived in London when I was arrested as a deserter from the Cape Peninsula Rifles of the South African Citizen Defence Force. The regiment, one gathered, was then under consideration for military service under General Smuts in East Africa against the Germans there. Through the good offices of the Honourable WP Schreiner, High Commissioner for the Union (of South Africa) in London, my desertion was condoned by General Smuts, no doubt with a smile, on the grounds that I was now on active service in a Territorial Regiment of the British army and destined shortly for the front line in Europe anyway.

'Many years later, when on the staff of the Johannesburg General Hospital, I learned one day that Major Maynard, then in the Public Health Service, had contracted streptococcal or pneumococcal meningitis and died in forty-eight hours. He was a fine officer and gentleman, typical of the English ruling classes of the day. A medical man with an exceptional breadth of mind and an advanced mathematical background, he played a conspicuous part in the epidemiological and statistical investigations that were then being undertaken by the State Health Service. While his batman in South-West Africa, I used to appreciate enormously the privilege and pleasure he gave me when, seated by the fireside on those starlit and cloudless cold tropical African nights, we used to discuss with much mutual satisfaction various higher mathematical concepts such as Stokes theorem and the like. It is said that it takes a gentleman to apologise, but I have always felt that my eventual apology to the Major for my atrocious terminal behaviour as his batman, lost much of its virtue by being coupled by a request for a testimonial to support enlistment in the British army. He was, of course, of too generous a nature to bear ill will, and sent me a kindly worded reference by return.'

I have quoted Craib freely in this vignette about the desert campaign seventy years ago in what is now often called Namibia, because it reveals a number of facets of his complex character: strong independence and decisive action when he considered his thinking to have been correct; early love of mathematics and the clarity of thought that it demands; occasional robust self-disparagement, possibly playful in tone; and scrupulous fairness in giving credit to his adversaries. These should be sought again and again in this account of the life of WH Craib and of his interpretation of the times in which he lived.

At war in Europe, 1915-1919

The intensity of the war in Europe, with its human carnage and its destruction of town and countryside alike, must have come as a shattering experience to Don Craib after the leisurely campaign in South-West Africa. In this respect he was undoubtedly like many other South Africans who fought in France and Belgium. Like some of them, he earned recognition for his conspicuous bravery—he was awarded the Military Cross and Bar and was twice mentioned in despatches—and he survived the war with lasting loyalties to his comrades-in-arms.

He was commissioned as a Second Lieutenant in the London Territorials at the end of 1915, but the urgent needs of the British Army for officers with a scientific or engineering background saw him transferred for gunnery training; so rapidly, in fact, that his first uniform was that of an officer in the Royal Field Artillery. The Somme offensive began in mid-1916 and the urgency of battle was so pressing that Craib found himself in France before he had experienced a live 'shoot' in training. He wrote that his first journey there was in a French railway truck marked '40 hommes et 8 cheveaux' which moved slowly but steadily towards 'the almost continuous booming roar of the guns and the flashes and flares that lit up the front line trenches at night'.

An inexperienced, train-dirty Craib found himself among guns emplaced and camouflaged in an apple orchard in the village of Engelbelmer. This battery was part of the Divisional Artillery of the 29th Division of the British Expeditionary Force. He was to become immensely proud of his membership of the '29th', but the impact of his early days in action, vividly remembered fifty years later, must have been varied and profound. He wrote that on the day of his arrival 'we fired at and were fired on by the German artillery opposite us, and I well recall the thrill of excitement when German shrapnel burst in our orchard without doing very much damage. Within a week I was sent up forward at night to learn something of the reserve and front line trench systems and to be introduced to the duties of forward observation officer. I recall my astonishment on finding during my first visit to the trenches, that the death of an infantryman killed by shrapnel at my side had no particular emotional effect upon me. *C'est la guerre*, and I, too, could expect to be killed or horribly broken at any moment of the day or night. I recall also my amazement when my battery commander one morning ordered me to see that his bathwater had been properly prepared, and my unspoken resentment that so menial a task should be put upon *me*. Shades of Major Maynard, and I began to wonder just how high or how low we colonials rated in the class distinctions of the British, or English, upper crust. In the mess at the Woolwich Gunnery School one had learnt something of the protocol, or proper bearing of an English officer and gentleman, but being ordered to prepare a senior officer's bath at the Front was indeed something else!'

A few weeks later Craib responded to an appeal for volunteers to serve in the Artillery Controlled Trench Mortar Batteries, the 'suicide brigade' as this branch of the service was colloquially known; partly, he said, to escape with honour from a commanding officer whom he could not admire. Here he remained throughout the war, becoming the sole survivor among his fellow mortar officers. Trained at a French mortar training school, he learnt short range trench artillery techniques and the use of hand grenades. Posted back to the 29th Division in the trenches on the river Aucre, his duties included observing where his battery's mortar shells exploded and reporting the position as accurately as possible by field telephone, so that the necessary adjustments could be made. He subsequently wrote that he was now 'hourly involved in the death and the dying and the agony of trench warfare, and on a scale that cannot be brought home to those who have never themselves been a part of it. Shells bursting a few yards away became a commonplace, and funerals at night an almost nightly chore. It was there that we watched the Black Watch in single file down Jacob's Ladder, in their kilts and thousands, taking up their battle positions at midnight preparatory to going over the top into a merciless spray of machine gun fire and shrapnel. Less than twelve hours later a mere 200 yards away was a writhing mass of wounded, dead and dying, unhelped and unhelpable till darkness protected their friends and stretcher bearers from snipers, if not from shells, bombs and machine gun bursts, that still kept taking their toll.'

Less than a month after his arrival his commanding officer was disembowelled by a howitzer shell outside their dugout; and he found himself in command of the battery. He retained this position until 1917 when Captain Booth, 'our magnificent and well loved Divisional Trench Mortars Commander' met a similar fate at the Battle of Cambrai. Craib succeeded him and remained in command until the end of the war eighteen months later, and for some time afterwards in the Army of Occupation.

In the fragments of his unpublished memoirs there are moving descriptions of several episodes involving Craib at war in the trenches. One of them, which merits quoting, he labelled 'Episode Rupert Brooke'.

'One cold Sunday afternoon in early 1917, lying on my back in a shellhole just beyond the Ypres Canal, enjoying the fitful sunshine, and waiting till it was dark enough to return to our dugout, I watched one of our RE8 (Harry Tab) biplanes slowly and monotonously flying overhead, up and down parallel to no-man's-land, and flashing back information to a rear area heavy battery as its shells burst in relation to its target deep in the Boche lines. Suddenly as I watched, the plane broke up in mid-air, obviously hit by a British shell on its way to the enemy. The pilot fell clear and plunged to earth some 50 yards from where I lay. I crawled out to see if there was anything to be done, but found him dead. Among his papers was a torn envelope containing a letter from his parents in Wales, dated some 7 days before.

'He was a young Welshman at work in the air, and in France for only about three weeks before his death. Scribbled on the envelope were the loosely written lines of a sonnet which read as follows:

> ". . . think only this of me; that there's some corner of a foreign field that is forever England . . ."

'The words impressed me so greatly that I could not help wondering whether they were original or taken from some published work. So I made a copy of them before returning his personal effects to his Unit, determined to find out their real origin.

'At that time I carried in my gas helmet container, an article one was never without, three small books, a *New Testament*, Plato's *Republic*, and . . . Housman's *Shropshire Lad.* I had also read something of Siegfried Sassoon's and was becoming interested in published poems by soldiers on active service, whenever a newspaper or journal of any kind came my way. The problem now was how to find out—whom to consult?'

His enquiries took him to a battery of territorials many of whose officers came from Warwickshire, 'an exceptionally delightful and erudite crowd of what I might describe as high quality minds'. Among them was John Eden, a cousin of Anthony Eden, and

Geoffrey Mure, who later became Dean of Merton College, Oxford. On his next home leave, Mure searched for the source of the fragment Craib had picked up and identified it as part of *The Soldier* by Rupert Brooke, who had died on active service in 1915.

On a wall in his study in Somerset East hung a composite picture of the salient beyond Ypres, put together from air reconnaisance maps. He described the map as showing 'British and German front line trenches facing each other in an area of unbelievable desolation, consisting solely of churned up mud and contiguous shell holes filled with water—probably the most revolting example of man's destructive ingenuity . . . before the atom bomb devastation at Hiroshima and Nagasaki'. Craib's mortar batteries were just behind the front line and he had made an arrow on the photograph suggesting where he might have been at the time. No-man's-land here was about 300 yards wide.

'One morning on observation duty', he wrote, 'wandering about in a lifting mist, I suddenly became aware of a lonely, half-frozen German infantryman disconsolately sitting in a shellhole, swinging his arms to keep warm and stamping his feet to avoid frost-bite. All we did was to take stock of each other in astonishment, remain dead still for a second, and then salute. I turned round and walked back into the mist. It was too cold to think of grabbing a weapon to shoot . . .'

'As Christmas approached the weather became colder, wetter, and mistier, and slush and snow added to the general discomfort. Front line troops on both sides were hard put to keep (free of) trench foot, frost-bite, and exhaustion collapse. The stretcher bearers, wounded and injured had a particularly bad time.

'By Christmas week human misery on both sides had reached (such) a pitch that by common consent mortar and machine gun firing had almost entirely ceased. One evening a number of Boche trench mortar bombs almost surprised us by their unfriendliness, but fell harmlessly if messily and noisily in the mud some 20 yards behind. The following morning our gunners walking about in no-man's-land in the mist, struggling to keep warm, heard a shouted apology from the enemy lines, saying, "Sorry, Tommy, but we had to shoot. Our officers had come with orders to fire. We hope our bombs fell beyond your positions into the mud behind." Which is of course just what they had done.

'On Christmas morn when the thick early morning mists were gently clearing, numbers of Germans and our own troops dimly discerned one another in no-man's-land, stamping up and down in parallel lines a hundred yards or less apart and swinging their arms to keep warm. They roared with laughter at their mutual predicament and shouted Christmas greetings to each other while a true Christmas spirit prevailed. As vision became clearer it became awkward, and both sides hopped back into their trenches once more.'

News of this fraternisation, greatly frowned upon by Divisional Command, led to a court martial of some fellow officers. Craib was summoned to give evidence at the enquiry. Those accused admitted that they were in no-man's-land on the morning in question but were unaware that there were Germans about; and Craib's evidence was that he heard no conversation between these particular officers and the enemy—sufficient, it would appear, to save the accused from penalties more severe than loss of a month's leave. In his memoirs Craib admitted that he had 'put up a poor performance in the eyes of the court'; he does not say whether he was asked if others had conversed with the Germans. Why they were punished at all, he wrote, was because they had failed to fire in order to kill as soon as they saw the enemy clearly enough to take aim.

As has been seen, Don Craib came from a deeply religious family. Elsewhere in this book will be recorded how involved he became with comparisons of statements about the same subject in various translations of the *Bible*. A tract from his memoirs which he entitled 'Carnage and Church' clearly shows how important religion was to him during the war. It also indicates the depth of his enquiring mind.

'To my friends,' he wrote, 'it might seem surprising, but to my intimates not so, when I say that religion is, in its broadest sense, of the very woof and warp of one's being. The relationship between man and his creator has been, I am sure, part of (my) thinking . . . every day of my life since about the age of ten. I am unable to look at the sky without pondering on the content of such words as infinity, Creator, God, Providence, Nature, nor at the earth without thinking of us, you, me, life in any of its multitudinous forms. Needless to say the almost daily experience of death during the active fighting phases of the Great War was not without its impact, causing one to cogitate unendingly in an effort to come to terms with such questions as why? how? whence? whither? and what is it all about?

'Where is it all going to end? . . . These millions, so suddenly and so ruthlessly slaughtered by forces over which they have no control, and which they cannot with any residual self respect avoid, so nobly doing their simple and patriotic duty . . . (are not) at least a percentage of these going to end up in eternal suffering and torment? Did Jesus of Nazareth not in effect bring salvation to all, saint and sinner alike! Of course there were the Army Chaplains of divergent denominations, periodically, if not at all times, available to preach to those of us whose duty it was on this occasion or that to attend a military church parade.

'As it happens I have always enjoyed the company of predikants, padres, priests, parsons, and rabbi and so not unnaturally took more interest than most of my fellow soldiers in the words, the prayers, the hymns and service patterns generally. Unconsciously perhaps I found myself particularly interested in the personality make-up of the clergy of the various denominations, their behaviour under fire, their empathy, their sincerity, their expressed views on sex, death, hellfire, belief, salvation and so on. Over the years one developed a partiality for clergymen of this denomination or that' . . . What appeared to impress him and the 'troops in the line, was not the power of their preaching, or the church ceremonials, but simply and solely the quietness of the man, his calm in danger, his readiness to share misery and discomfort, and his easy availability and infectious cheerfulness when needed by the sick, the wounded and the dying. My highest regard in France and Flanders was awarded to Anglican padres and Roman Catholic priests.

'We in the Artillery were extremely blessed in an Army Chaplain, the Reverend JW Hunkin—or plain Hunks as his many friends and admirers generally called him. A Cambridge man, of Gonville and Caius College, he was small in stature but a giant in kindliness, friendliness, sincerity, unfailing energy, and, as was obvious to all, completely lacking in fear at all times. His texts were usually taken from Biblical stories of brave and unselfish men, and never but never did he lash us with stories of impending torment. All of us felt somehow that old Hunks would be there to plead for us on the Day of Judgement, and that because of his pleadings, things might not turn out so badly after all.

'Hunks had a curious almost naive habit of turning up unexpectedly at the hottest point of the battle, bearing on his back a haversack—full of fags, chocolates, pain killers and other goodies—

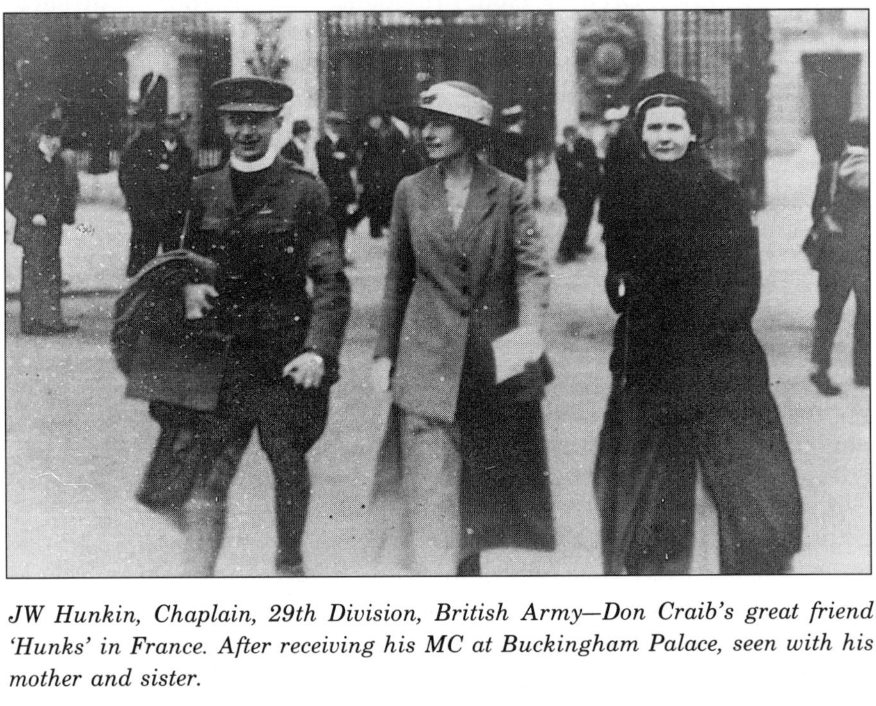

JW Hunkin, Chaplain, 29th Division, British Army—Don Craib's great friend 'Hunks' in France. After receiving his MC at Buckingham Palace, seen with his mother and sister.

that became almost an insignia of his military contribution. Although a cleric, he was almost as deeply concerned with human happiness as with spiritual comfort. The effect of his words at a funeral service in the line—and he must have buried hundreds, almost where they died—was one of calm and peacefulness. He developed a habit, almost undisciplined it might be said, of being in hot spots where he had no right to be.'

One of the closest friendships Don Craib developed at the front was with this Anglican priest. With only his clerical collar and his lack of arms to distinguish him from others, Hunks would appear in the fighting lines at any time of day or night for a friendly chat, his way of bringing moral and spiritual support. On one occasion Don met up with him when both dived into a shellhole in no-man's-land, whither they had wandered separately during a lull in the fighting. Before either could speak, all hell was let loose by the enemy and as soon as the shelling ceased—as abruptly as it had begun—both left hurriedly for other destinations without uttering a word. On another, during a hand-to-hand midnight skirmish, his commanding officer, Major Booth was killed and Craib taken prisoner. He was led under guard to a cellar where, to his surprise, he found Hunks in a similar predicament. 'When I laughingly questioned him about the irregularity of his presence in the front line areas, he replied that he had been asked to visit a forward casualty clearing station with a message to the effect that if the Germans were likely to capture it, would the medicals kindly remove certain essential gadgets from all serviceable vehicles in order to prevent their being used by the enemy. The clearing station in mind had already been captured by the Boche, and Hunks merely walked into the enemy hands, where I subsequently joined him.' Their captors, recently arrived from the Russian front, had apparently been informed that the war in the west was all but over; they were therefore shocked to find how intense was the fighting. Before long they said they were tired of the war and wished to give themselves up to the British. Prisoners and captors changed places; 'so we picked up the wounded, both British and German, and silently filed back through a sort of no-man's-land in the general direction of our own battered front line'.

In many ways Hunks and Don were kindred spirits. Joseph Wellington Hunkin first came up to Cambridge to read mathematics, entering Caius College in 1906 and gaining a first each year. After graduating he turned to the theology tripos. In the First World War he served with distinction as chaplain in the 29th Division in Gallipoli and in France, where he and Craib became friends. Each, no doubt, admired the other's warmth of personality, intellectual gifts and conspicuous bravery. By the end of the war, each had twice been mentioned in despatches and had gained the MC and Bar. Hunkin became Dean at Caius immediately after the war and later

Tutor in Theology, serving the College for many years until he moved on, eventually becoming Bishop of Truro in 1935. After his death in 1950, a moving tribute to his bravery was paid to him by the Warden of Merton College, Oxford. Writing in *The Times*, he described his dedication to duty as chaplain and his fearlessness in the front line, ending with the words: 'We loved him much as a hero, much as a very human saint, and perhaps a little as a mascot'. He was described as an outstanding pastoral bishop in *The Caian*, the Caius College journal, recording that 'it was the sheer goodness of the man which enabled his interest in the working of men's minds and emotions to be used to the great comfort of his people and the greater glory of God'. As a theologian, he was a modernist in his views: perhaps, like Craib, a bit of a rebel. And Craib would have liked Hunkin's belief that the creeds needed restatement; in their present wording they could 'only be accepted with considerable liberty of interpretation'. No wonder Don so loved the man.

There were other episodes which Craib must have found amusing. In one of them he records how he was joined at a forward observation post by a group of British officers. His own task as usual was to report back how his battery's mortar shells were landing in relation to their target. The other officers were the first to register how their shells had landed. Craib told them his own mortar shells were not as reliable as theirs, often falling short and as such were a distinct danger; he firmly suggested that they withdraw, a suggestion they treated with contempt. 'To my dismay nobody accepted my advice to move', he wrote. 'In fact they refused to lose so exceptional an opportunity to see a heavy trench mortar bomb bursting a mere 150 yards away on the enemy front line. If I didn't take my own advice, they said, why the this and that should they? As it was the enemy had been unusually quiet all night and during their shoot, and all the omens therefore seemed pleasantly propitious. So I gave the order to fire, and the first bombs passed high over our heads detonating with a tremendous roar on the enemy line ahead. We all turned to watch the third bomb leave the cellar about 200 yards to the rear. It duly appeared in impressive style, but seemed a bit slow to my trained eye, and one feared the worst. Suddenly one of the watchers gave a startled yell to the effect that the damn(ed) thing was going to fall on us. "Yes", I said "it's going to fall short, so all you chaps better lie damn flat in the mud, it's your only hope now." The bomb entered the ground some 30 yards away in the midst of a collection of two-gallon petrol cans filled with water preparatory to the advance. For what seemed an eternity nothing happened and I thought "that's, thank goodness, a dud". Suddenly the earth opened in an almighty explosion, petrol cans, tree stumps, stones and earth and mud flew in all directions, and everybody lay still till the fall of debris subsided. Suddenly the prostrate earth worshippers in their mud-drenched uniforms, realising that they were still alive and unhurt, got up and stood not upon the order of their going. Indeed I had hardly recovered my own equilibrium before I realised that all around was dead silence, a man of corruption, and not a soul in sight.'

Craib must have enjoyed recalling this story for he always regarded himself as a 'colonial'; he was perhaps more conscious than most young English-speaking men and women from the old Dominions of feeling inferior (and in Craib's case, with very little cause) when face to face with what he used to call the 'English upper crust'. From what he wrote he clearly had in mind his South African accent, its Eastern Cape origins obvious in later years only to a discerning ear. He also records that 'to us colonials, Britons in matters of what's "done" and "not done" were, by and large, an unpredictable crowd. Delightfully casual about some things, they could be unshakeably addicted to others, a variation in behaviour patterns that derived from wide deviations in cultural class practices.'

He developed the highest admiration for what he called the military officer class, particularly their deep sense of honour and their bravery. But he was obviously amused and probably carried some hurt from his early days of officer training in England when he wrote that not to conform strictly to protocol 'after or during dinner in mess, (by) smoking before the King's health (was proposed) . . . was indubitable proof of the low social class of one's (background)'. He manifestly relished his own story of being entertained by a fellow artillery officer 'in an abandoned pill box . . . his guns in emplacements surrounded by mud and filth and sandbags, just beyond the Boesinghe canal. Mine host was a great stickler for the niceties of traditional Woolwich grammar school behaviour under all circumstances if at all possible. We even had specially preserved and highly prized wine glasses on display. The table was composed of ammunition boxes about 18 inches high, covered with a cloth, round which we sat in a sideways position, almost greedily staring at one or two goodies of Fortnum and Mason origin. Time came when a fag seemed indicated, but we had of course first to toast His Majesty the King. To do so required a physical manoeuvre that amuses me to this day. The toast had to be drunk standing, requiring our legs in an extended position and our spine(s) at right angles horizontally. I've just attempted to repeat the performance and had to smile at the accompanying arthritic creaks!'

Craib's obvious amusement about some of the behaviour patterns of his fellow officers in the British Army in the First World War has a ring about it that makes it similar to what colonials from the old British Empire and many Americans often expressed. Their British counterparts in both world wars no doubt had just as much fun, and indulged in as much criticism, about English-speakers from outside the United Kingdom. What comes through quite clearly, however, is the deep admiration Craib developed for what he called

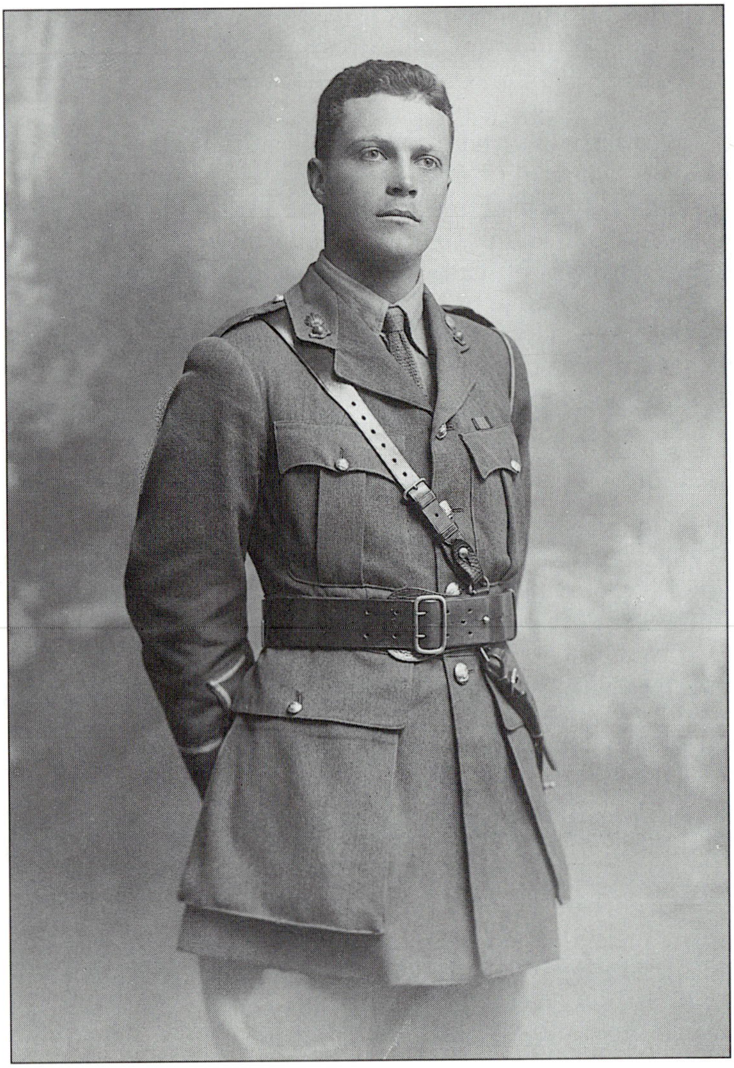

A/Capt WH Craib, MC & Bar, Trench Mortar Officer, 29th Division, British Army, France 1915–1918.

the 'British officer class': admiration which only soured fifty years later over the Rhodesian independence issue.

Don Craib seldom spoke of his military honours but must have felt deep pride in his bravery. Seeking information for their archives, the South African Council for Scientific and Industrial Research in 1973 obtained details about his MC from the British Ministry of Defence. The record obtained from the Army Medal Office, Droitwich, reads as follows:

Lt (A/Capt) William Hofmeyr Craib, RFA:
-Awarded Military Cross London Gazette 1 Jan. 1918.
-Awarded Bar to Military Cross London Gazette 4 Feb. 1918.

No citation was available for the first of these but for the Bar the citation was:

> 'For conspicuous gallantry and devotion to duty. With another officer he organized a party of infantry, and himself led a counter-attack which drove the enemy out of the village. He then advanced further, and came upon a party of the enemy at very close quarters. The other officer was wounded, but he maintained a determined resistance, and succeeded in driving back the enemy. It was entirely due to the efforts of these two officers that an advanced dressing station was recaptured.'

Don was to be reminded of this or a similar episode many years later in a letter received from Major Charles Ball, written from his farm in Hampshire in March 1969. The Balls and the Craibs had planned a holiday in France which had been cancelled. 'I was really looking forward', Major Ball wrote, 'to visiting the Cambrai area again, with you, and seeing if we could find the house from which you and Hunks brought away the wounded, with "Bosch" machine guns firing overhead. And finding some of your TM Battery positions on the Somme, or at Arras . . .'

Like many others, Don Craib's friendships made in war were to be treasured for the rest of his life.

Chapter 3

Cambridge and Guy's

Early in 1919, Craib went up to Cambridge to study medicine.

I found among his papers a charming memoir which reflects what he must have felt in the peace and tranquility of this lovely East Anglian city after the death and destruction of the war. In it he recounts an interview with the Senior Tutor at Trinity, the college which he had set his heart upon while still at school. The story was retold many times in after years, often differing in detail but never in substance, so it is probably a fair version of how he became an undergraduate at Caius College. Like so many of his tales, there may have been some fantasy mixed with the truth: an accusation to which he would certainly have taken exception, granting how deeply he felt about truth! But the recounting of past events by most of us surely has a built-in variability, no matter how slight, so that fact and fancy mingle.

Still in uniform and 'looking fairly respectable and far less shabby than four weeks later', Craib was asked by the Senior Tutor (who had already perused his letters and other admission documents) why he had chosen Trinity. Craib replied that he had always wished to come up to Trinity, even in his school days, and had had South African friends there, like Oliver Schreiner; and he added (no doubt in a Puckish way) that there had been trouble with Germany which had cost him five years, so he would like to be admitted immediately. Impossible, he was told, there were too many other soldiers returning from the war; his name would go on a waiting list for possible admission in six months' time. Craib wrote the rest of the account as follows:

> Craib: 'Sir, if you were in my shoes, what would you do?'
> Senior Tutor: 'I'm afraid I also would think six months a long time to wait.'
> Craib: 'Then, Sir, don't you think I should seek entry to another college in Cambridge?'
> Senior Tutor (looking very surprised): 'Dear, dear! what an odd question! Is there another college do you think?'
> Craib (smiling broadly): 'I think I know what you mean, Sir, but you know better than I do. Won't you please recommend one?'
> Senior Tutor (thinking hard): 'Well now, let me see!' (scratches his head) 'You know, I've heard a rumour recently that there is a college somewhere in that direction,' indicating with his thumb over his shoulder. 'Why not try that?'

A few minutes later he was told by the porter in the college next door how to find the Senior Tutor. But on the way, 'gazing at the beauty of Tree Court in the early spring', he met Padre Hunkin—'old Hunks of the 29th' —now Dean of the College, who arranged his admission and a little later even contrived to assist Craib in his relative penury by awarding him a small stipend for help in chapel.

And so Don Craib became a member of Gonville and Caius College.

Writing later about 'the happy bond between the College Dean, old Hunks' and himself, a bond never spoken of during Hunkin's lifetime, Craib recounted how his stipend had come about. 'I cannot help smiling when I recall the occasion during the early days at Caius when he invited me to have breakfast in his rooms above the Gate of Virtue. "Look, Don," he said, "I need some help—perhaps you'll come to my rescue. I often hold services in the early morning—I might almost say its a statutory duty for me to do so as part of my job—and no one turns up, especially when its cold and raining, or just too beautiful a day to waste indoors. You see, I need a congregation to make the responses and someone to read the lessons—or do a few odd things that have to be done before as well as during the service. Won't you please take on the job, at a stipend of £ 25 a term?" (Or it might have been a year, I forget.) Of course I was delighted to "help" him, and equally of course he did it only to help me; but being the gentleman he was, he didn't know quite how to offer me money without referring to my rather pathetic financial situation.' In later life, Don used to say, with a twinkle in his eye, that he was Organ Scholar at Caius College, Cambridge.

'What happy days those were', he wrote. 'Actually at Cambridge at last, even if not at Trinity. Slowly adapting to a "gentleman's life". The freedom of it, the safety of it, the comfort and cleanliness of it after those filthy years of mud and slush and the stench of death. Poling a punt to Granchester to see the village clock at ten to three, immortalised by Rupert Brooke before he died so tragically at war. Dozing on a summer's day in the lush green grass beside the Granta and surrounded by innumerable yellow buttercups. The woods alive with bluebells close by. Men sitting silently for hours on the river bank with their inevitable rod to catch an unsuspecting perch or pole or pike or two—poor pike! Lovely English girls gracefully at ease on brightly coloured cushions in newly varnished punts, while their thrice lucky swains gently poled their ungainly craft upstream. The loud musical note or chirrup of English birds in the willows. The slow stirring of heart and mind to resist the call of "dolce far niente" and to rediscipline its habit to the serious matter of the storing of knowledge. The burning of midnight oil. The terror that perhaps one has lost forever the ability to concentrate on lectures, tutorials and textbooks, an aptitude that had, in seemingly prehistoric times, enabled one to separate and to hoard for future use, the wheat from the chaff in one's reading. The simple pleasure of an evening's entertainment watching a play from the cheap and crowded, uncomfortable seats in the pit of the local theatre. The deep spiritual and intellectual satisfactions that stirred one's deepest magics as one sat at the feet of men of the calibre of RA Peters, now world famous as Sir Rumbold Peters of Oxford; Sir Gowland Hopkins, who was busy inventing vitamins; (Adrian) the physiologist, now Lord Adrian in the House of Lords. The dinners in Hall. The new kind of talk at all hours of the night in each other's rooms. And all of it still on a high clean note of almost adolescent rededication to go on doing something good in the world. The unconscious shedding of the spiritual slime of years of indescribable filthy death or loss of limb—all cast off like a soiled garment. One's mind and body cleansed forever in the healing ambient promise of lovely things to be because we had conquered in a war against all that is foul in the relationship of one man or nation and another. A free new world had been born from fire and blood and we were alive and in it! A world for which so many millions had suffered or died or both—so unprotestingly, so violently, so filthily. I weep as I write, for it really was so.

'Never again shall countless young men march side by side into a spray of lead, to fall wounded or dead across coils of uncut barbed wire entanglements, which their comrades, the field and trench mortar gunners, had failed to disperse so that they might pass unhindered. Millions of us—French, British, Colonials, Indians, Germans, Russians, Americans too in the end, dying inextricably and inexplicably at the call of patriotism and loyalty, convinced of the good and sometimes the God for which and for whom they were so willing to die.

'But at Cambridge, as at Oxford and elsewhere, the young and not so young, ourselves, were about to enter, if not the millenium, at least something pretty close to it. An era characterised by integrities that would replace for all time the still discernible strands of spiritual filth that have trailed from man ever since he emerged from his primordial slime. We were convinced, or had persuaded ourselves, that the war to end war had been fought and won. We knew, like the Jews of old, that we too had entered a promised land on 11th November, 1918.

'Now at the age of twenty-five, or thereabouts, we worked and swotted and listened and wrote and memorised like small boys at school avid to grow up into men. We sat next to grown men who looked like boys, just up from school in the first flush of 'Varsity. They never seemed to work, yet always had the answers and headed the lists. With them we had no conversation for we had nothing in common. We drifted around in ex-army groups, tremblingly conscious of the enchanting beauty of young womanhood in the tea shops and parks and women's colleges, Newnham and Girton. We withheld ourselves from their company, afraid of premature involvement. We were shy to make friends for we could hold out no promise, all energy and savings to be reserved for the years ahead of study and training. Those College dances where pre-war formalism was being replaced by a new drawing together, a getting closer. The ballroom fears that one might be creating a wrong and unlovely impression by pressing too close to enticing loveliness.

'Reading *The New Psychology* by Tansley, I think it was, *Sinister Street* by Compton McKenzie, *The Green Hat* and something of the new philosophies. Meeting the Higher Criticism, standing in deep emotional and architectural admiration before or within the old churches and ancient cathedrals of the British Isles. Learning to sense the as yet undiscovered and unexplained strange traditional beliefs, mannerisms, behaviour patterns of the different racial groups, almost tribal in their stark divergence, of the peoples of Britain, the Welsh, Scots, the English, the Irish—no longer brothers in arms of different accents and strange vocabularies; no longer one large family of fighting men with a common enemy to destroy or be destroyed. Slowly awakening to the fact that the clear and shining target was daily becoming more and more deeply enshrouded in mist, old thoughts being replaced by new thoughts. "Just what had it all been about or for?" "Where did Christianity come in?" "Just what is patriotism, anyway?"

'But why waste time, we said, upon such extraneous and controversial considerations when one had a living to earn and only a small savings account to cover the expensive but necessary training? Indeed, to which of the famous hospitals in the great cities of Britain should one apply for admission became a burning question as the finals of our non-clinical years drew nigh. Above all, which could I afford?

'At Caius, and indeed Cambridge, there were no ordinary opportunities for riotous living and no need therefore publicly to cut one's coat according to one's cloth. My relative penury remained unspotted. Gossip had it that a London hospital was a sine qua non to professional success. St Thomas's and Bart's were highly favoured; Guy's was said to be far too surgically slanted, while Middlesex and the rest were either too small or undesirable for this reason or that. All nonsense, of course, but that was the talk.'

Craib was clearly worried by his finances. He believed that his wealthier friends would go to St Thomas's or Bart's and thought that few of his friends would be going to Guy's. So he chose Guy's Hospital and remarked what a lucky choice it turned out to be.

He must have left Cambridge with many regrets but richer in his experiences and in the many friendships he made there. Among them was the Master of Caius, Dr Anderson*—'quite the kindest and most gentle of men'—who left him his Doctor of Medicine gown, which

*Sir Hugh Kerr Anderson, Master 1912–1928.

Craib valued highly, for it remained in his wardrobe until his death. 'Why (he left it to me) I never knew and never shall', he jotted down in a scrap-book in 1969. But being remembered in this way is not altogether surprising, for Craib's intellectual gifts must have impressed Dr Anderson and some, at least, of the Fellows of the College. 'There was at one time', he wrote in the same memoir, 'some talk of my one day becoming a Fellow of Caius, the highest honour a college has to bestow. But with the background of war and a Calvinistic upbringing, I felt I could not let myself ease out from my obligations to mankind, however honourably, by quietly floating away into so utterly delectable a backwater as a college fellowship at that time appeared to be. There was an urge to get on with living that would not be gainsaid.' It is perhaps of some interest to record in this study of the man that Craib had scrawled across the cover of the scrap-book the words: 'I write for myself. Private conversations. A haphazard affair.'

At Cambridge, too, he began a lifelong association with another South African, Basil Schonland, who later married Craib's sister Ismay, then up at Newnham on a scholarship: both of them highly intelligent. His sister Ismay, he wrote, 'was the brainy member of our family. I always pictured her as achieving fame through her writings in an historical context, and possibly novels in the style of CP Snow. But she has devoted her talents and her life to the support and comfort of a great man, her husband, and has had no time left over for original contributions of her own.' For Basil Schonland was to achieve fame for his researches in the fields of lightning, radar and nuclear physics, become a Fellow of the Royal Society, succeed Sir John Cockcroft as Director of Harwell, and be honoured by a knighthood.

Craib wrote this about Schonland: 'A brilliant physicist with a brilliant war record during which he was responsible for research that improved military communications on active service, he and I at one stage shared rooms . . . (These) had once been lived in by Dr Wilson, who died at the South Pole on that most tragic of expeditions when Oates walked out of the tent to die, rather than endanger the lives of his fellow explorers by holding them back in a race against time. His feet were too badly frozen to walk . . . Basil was knighted for his work on atomic physics and lightning. I have a feeling that Cockcroft and Basil and perhaps Penney too were all workers with Rutherford at the Cavendish at Cambridge during the fantastic contributions of that laboratory to our present day understanding of nuclear physics.'

These two passages from his writings draw attention once again to two of Craib's characteristics: his generosity about the achievements of others, even when they were as close to him as his sister and his brother-in-law; and his deep admiration of bravery. There is no doubt about his feelings for Basil Schonland on both of these scores. His distinguished career as a scientist is recorded in the *Biographical Memoirs of Fellows of The Royal Society,* and as regards his bravery, he was twice mentioned in dispatches and decorated OBE, Military Division in the First World War. Moreover, in several fields of operation in World War 2 his service was equally distinguished. Eventually, as Brigadier Schonland, he became scientific adviser to General Montgomery with the Army of Liberation and decorated again. The award was the CBE(Mil) for services at the battle of Caen, the citation reading 'in recognition of gallant and distinguished services in the field'.

After Cambridge, being a clinical student in London and living in lodgings near Guy's Hospital clearly entailed considerable adjustments. It was, Craib wrote, 'somewhat of a change from Cambridge. Instead of living as a monk in College with periodic immersion in the beauty of the countryside, one now sheltered rather than lived in a simple room in digs not far removed from slums. That was all one could afford. A bed-sitter it was called; first in Trinity Square, and then at the Pig and Whistle. No bathroom and little more than a bed and chest of drawers, with a mat on the floor that looked encrusted, shall I say. A single suitcase held the glad-rags left over from Cambridge—and which, alas, one was too poor to sport.' During training in midwifery, his accommodation was better because he lodged in the 'College' built across the street from the hospital, mainly for housemen and registrars. It appears that Ryle (later Sir John Ryle) was the member of staff in charge. Ryle, Craib wrote, 'was at the time slowly but meticulously building up a consulting practice in the famous and notorious Wigmore Street or Harley Street areas of London' on his way to achieving great distinction in his career. Perhaps his use of the word 'notorious' reflected some of the popular writings of the day.

Craib was always a disciplined letter-writer, composing them with commendable economy. They were invariably clear and to the point, and often couched in warm terms. Judging by the number of drafts of letters found in his study after his death, many of them differing from the previous one mainly in the language he had used, he made quite sure that his meaning was unambiguous. His letters often commenced with a light-hearted salutation and might include a playful leg-pull or an amusing anecdote. During the mid-1920s, while he was away in England and the United States, Don Craib wrote weekly letters to his parents at their home in Somerset East, many of which have been preserved. Some are worth quoting because they help to throw light on his early life and on his attitudes about his home and his close-knit family.

'Your mail letter this week', he wrote from London late in 1924, 'brought its usual welcome breath of African air to a very drab, dingy corner of the globe—namely Bermondsey. It's always a red letter day—Monday.' He must have written this while staying with friends, for the address was 8 Queensberry Place, SW, the home in Kensington of AH Wilson, who had entertained Craib and many other officers on leave from France during the war, and continued to do so later. Having completed his years of clinical training as a medical student at Guy's Hospital and obtained his medical degree, he was working in the hospital as a junior doctor. He had had 'a long day of babies, fractures, skins, coughs, colds, throats and all the other things that fill an out-patient officer's day'. Nostalgia for Gardiol and a longing for news of the doings of his family comes through clearly in this letter—as indeed it does in most of his letters home over the next three years.

A few months later he wrote about his work in the wards at Guy's. That day two young men had died from lobar pneumonia—one a South African dental student and the other a professional cricketer. 'These two heavy cases plus the usual work, including a very sick hospital nurse and a . . . doctor, made our hands pretty full, especially at night. So today I feel like the Gardiol stoep in a deck chair for at least a fortnight!' This and many subsequent letters from both London and Baltimore included many brief references to his home and his sisters Ismay and Dot. He often wrote about his brothers Murray and Ian, with whom he had close friendships. From time to time he would meet up with one or the other while they too were studying in Britain or the United States. They clearly had a lot of fun together; but his letters also showed his caring attitude and his concern for their welfare and success in their careers in radiology and forestry. Sincere interest in what others were doing became a striking characteristic of Don Craib's and many will remember him for this side of his warm personality.

Not much is known about his years as a clinical student and a resident doctor at Guy's Hospital, but he must have distinguished himself because it was while he was there that he was nominated for and awarded a Rockefeller Fellowship. This is generally held in high regard by the medical profession. More information about his career at Guy's and the circumstances of this award, as he saw them, comes from his scrap-book. 'What interests me most in looking back is the quality of the experience and training and teaching one received in order to qualify for professional practice. The emphasis was on diagnosis and technique in both medical and surgical wards, with almost complete absence of theory. If one couldn't solve a problem, why let it bother you? The theory of medicine was in those days at an unimpressive stage with very little in the way of evidence. Experiments on man himself, except in surgery, had as yet had no particular impact on the treatment of the sick . . . Strange as it may seem, it is nevertheless true that in the early days of the second decade of this century, we doctors could do marvels of cure with the knife but almost nothing at all with the potion or the pill. I can remember quinine for malaria, emetine for amoebic dysentery, iron for housemaid's anaemia, strawberries for sprue, and leeches for pericarditis . . . ' And here in his memoirs his sense of mischievous fun surfaced with the added remark about leeches that in the examination for the Membership of the Royal College of Physicians of London (a most sought-after postgraduate qualification), 'this suggestion . . . I am sure, so impressed the more ancient of my examiners that their thumbs were involuntarily moved from a downward to an upward position'.

His scrap-book also shows that Don Craib made many friends. One was AH Wilson, an elderly London solicitor who was a cousin of a Scots woman known to the Craib family in Somerset East. During the war she would send him the names of 'Somerset boys' or others serving in the British Army; and he in turn made a point of inviting them to dine or to stay at his home in Kensington while they were on leave. 'A letter from Mr Wilson reached me on the Somme and I spent my first leave after about twelve months of trench warfare' at his obviously elegant home. For it was here, he continued, that he saw his first work by a distinguished artist (Rosa Bonheur), had his first claret cup and enjoyed, for the first time, good French and German wines. Through Wilson's hospitality, too, he began to appreciate ballet and opera at Covent Garden and theatre in the West End—in particular, Bernard Shaw. He was also invited 'for meals or for weekends at the houses of what in those days might be referred to as the creme de la creme, the upper class gentry—who spent their lives huntin', ridin' and fishin'; born, all of them, with a silver spoon in their mouths. Anyone who has read Sarah Gertrude Millin's *Goodbye Dear England* will know exactly what I mean—she described London and England during the '14–'18 War years with an extraordinarily unerring touch. When I read the description of London in those days, I relive my experiences at 8 Queensberry Place.'

He also wrote of others whom he recalled 'with enormous affection', like Sir Edward Boland and his wife Barbara, who were then living in retirement in their charming home in Kent. Boland had enlisted in 1915 when he was a medical student at Guy's. He was only seventeen when he volunteered for combatant service and had shown 'quite fantastic dedication and sacrifice in World War 1,' (from which) 'he emerged sans eye, sans kidney, and (with) ghastly wounds to arms and legs'. Nevertheless, he resumed his medical studies at Guy's in 1918 and was to spend most of his professional life there, eventually becoming one of the senior physicians and Dean. They were to meet again in Rome and in Cairo during the Second World War when Boland held high military rank. Through him, Craib had an audience with the Pope. He was a few years ahead of Craib at medical school and it is clear that there was a lasting bond of friendship between them. As recorded in *Munk's Roll* at the Royal College of Physicians, London, 'his innate kindness and the respect and courtesy he displayed to his patients set an example to his junior staff that was difficult to emulate', qualities which Don must have admired as much as Boland's distinguished war record.

For the purposes of this book, Dr John Conybeare must rank as the most important of the many who befriended him. The author of a textbook of medicine used by generations of medical students in the English-speaking world, Conybeare was a junior physician at Guy's when Craib was a student. Many years later Don recalled that he 'took great interest in helping young men to enlarge themselves outside as well as inside medicine. Many a young colonial was taken by Cony in his Studebaker and a succession of Morrises . . . for 48-hour rambles midst the beauty of the countryside anything up to 60–70 miles from London.'

In *Munk's Roll*, among Conybeare's many qualities and distinctions, which included a Military Cross for his bravery and resourcefulness on the Somme, I found the following passage: 'A radical, both by lineage and conviction, while remaining a believer in authority, he nevertheless was a supporter of the underdog. He could be a thorn in the flesh of the administrator; he would brook no delay in bringing to notice any case where he suspected injustice.' Later on it will be seen that some of these characteristics may also be attributed to Craib, who clearly liked him. Conybeare must have sized up Craib's intellectual worth, for it was he who put his young colleague's name forward for a Rockefeller Fellowship. Craib described this as follows:

> 'Towards the end of my houseman or internship year, with no private means for postgraduate training, and nothing but an assistantship in private practice looming ahead, Dr Conybeare stopped me one day and said, quite out of the blue, 'How would you like to do research in the USA on a Rockefeller grant?' Convinced that he must be joking or addressing the question to someone else, I quickly glanced round. But no, it was really to me that he had put the question.
>
> 'My career at Guy's had been about as humdrum as any average medical student's performance could be. More than that, my Calvinistic upbringing, my university education devoted entirely to the mathematical sciences, followed by five years in unbroken active service of which nearly 3 had been spent in a trench mortar unit in the trenches in France and Flanders, and finally the usual elementary preclinical studies as provided at Cambridge, had left me with a sort of dormant and unscientific imagination as though dogmas were infallible, and conformity the quickest way to security.
>
> 'And then Conybeare's question—like manna from heaven! But how could I, unfitted as I knew myself to be, accept so incredible, so momentous an offer and yet retain my self respect? Would I

not be a charlatan, an imposter—accepting money to which I could produce no single claim?'

Sir John Conybeare, as he later became, had himself been at the Johns Hopkins Hospital, Baltimore, on a Rockefeller Fellowship, and Don Craib must have overcome his scruples, for the late summer of 1925 found him on his way to the same great institution in the United States. 'Truly someone had rubbed Aladdin's lamp', he wrote, 'and the Holy Grail was mine. It was an act of generosity on Conybeare's part that astonishes me to this day.' If Craib's self-denigration of his student career is taken at face value, Conybeare must be credited as having been a remarkable judge of human potential!

In his scrap-book Don wrote: 'It took eight days to cross the ocean, four seasick in bed, and four in saloon or on deck under the wet grey skies of the North Atlantic. Two charming American girl tourists for some queer reason of their own took charge of me, one of them calling me her 'little white wabbit'—which rather shook an intrepid trench-mortarman not long out of the trenches, nor yet the hero of even the mildest of one of those nurse-medical student skirmishes that are said to open the eyes of young men in metropolitan medical schools to the more startling facts of life.'

Don Craib was met at the docks in New York by his brother Ian, and they soon went off together to see Yale, where Ian was working, and the Niagara Falls. A letter home from Baltimore showed how much the two of them had enjoyed this jaunt; it also made it obvious that he found Baltimore to his liking for 'there are many things here that remind one of South Africa and home. Sweet potatoes, mealies, melons, grapes, pumpkins in the food line—and the climate and type of house are also very suggestive.'

So began his year at Johns Hopkins. It was here that he was to make a significant contribution to medical science by carrying out research which was surprisingly simple in design and execution, and which in turn would lead to the first of several major controversies which characterised his brilliant career.

Chapter 4

Craib's Doublet Hypothesis

Don Craib arrived in Baltimore in the late summer of 1925 on a coveted fellowship from the Rockefeller Foundation. His first letter home from the United States revealed how impressed he was by the large full-time medical staff at Johns Hopkins Hospital (in comparison with Guy's where the consultant staff were usually honorary). He also remarked that there were many young medical graduates, like himself, working as research fellows on clinical or physiological research projects. He found the atmosphere distinctly academic—unlike at Guy's where 'everything is looked at from the purely practical point of view'. What he also found particularly impressive at Johns Hopkins was the generous supply of electrical and other equipment for research.

In his first venture into medical research, Craib worked in the laboratories directed by Dr EP Carter. Many years later one of Don's new Baltimore friends, Dr E Cowles Andrus, sent him a memorial note about Carter which he had written for the Interurban Clinical Club. He described his commanding stature (six foot four) and his good humour, remarking on his 'subtle, entertaining wit' and his 'obvious distaste for pretentiousness and aggressiveness'. At his best teaching at the bedside, he was a most competent and thoughtful physician, communicating effectively 'to those about him an understanding of the opportunities and obligations to learn from the sick person about disease and (gain) insight into the purpose and significance of research'. Craib's sort of man, it might be added, Carter clearly had a tremendous influence on Don's life-long conviction that clinical practice must be allied to clinical research, accepted beliefs being continually challenged and put to the test.

In the stimulating environment of Johns Hopkins Hospital, Don soon found himself challenging the accepted beliefs about electrical fields created by active heart muscle. Within a few months he had written home that 'things are going very well but it remains to be seen how long this happy state of affairs will continue'. His prewar training in mathematics at the university in Cape Town, he said, stood him in good stead, for his research colleagues were 'physiologists pure and simple and the physiologist's idea of physics is a rather hazy affair (and) unfortunately for them modern physiological research requires greatly wider pure science knowledge than in years gone by . . . '

Many years later he recalled that he was immediately confronted in the wards of the hospital by the phenomenon of cardiac electricity—not as an abstract theory but as a practical fact that was invaluable in the management of the sick. Electrocardiology was being developed in the United States with great benefit for the study of heart disease, and he was immediately 'consumed with a desire to know all there was to be known about electricity originating in living cells'. His attention was drawn to a scientific monograph published in England and written by Sir Thomas Lewis, who was widely regarded at the time as the world authority on electrocardiological theory. Craib came to the subject 'with an open mind, unprejudiced and untutored and . . . a nonentity'. As he read the explanations of how living tissue like heart muscle produced recordable electrical currents, he found himself at sea. It seemed to him that the electrophysiologists of 1925 drew a distinction between the electricity of the engineering world with which he was familiar, and electricity generated by living tissues: a belief he totally rejected. Craib put it this way: 'Either the physicists of 1913, or the electro-cardiologists of 1925, were mistaken. They could both be wrong, but certainly they could not both be right *unless*, indeed, there were two kinds of electricity at work in the world, one associated with living organs, the other to be found only in inanimate matter.' He rejected this possibility, reasoning that in the final analysis living tissues are themselves composed of nothing but a conglomeration of inanimate particles.

He was consumed with curiosity to find the truth behind this apparent paradox. With Dr Carter's concurrence, he designed several simple experiments to test what he described as 'a few elementary principles obtainable only from direct observation'. He was behaving in this respect precisely as he did throughout his life, displaying both a measure of humility and a clarity of thought that set him apart from most of his fellows. More than forty years later, writing about his Johns Hopkins experience, he recalled that he had 'never done research before but . . . did have at the back of his mind the conviction that the only truth is fact, that fact is something that can be observed and recorded, and that all that we do when we attempt to explain a fact or a truth, in terms of this wordy principle or that, consists of nothing but theory, guess, hypothesis, supposition, assumption, postulate or conjecture'.

His first study involved the freshwater tortoise. Immediately after sacrificing this reptile, the heart was removed intact and suspended in Ringer's saline. The heart continued to beat regularly or could be stimulated to do so. Two non-polarisable electrodes connected to a sensitive galvanometer were placed at various positions in relation to the heart. 'When both electrodes were several inches distant from the beating heart no deflections were observed on this galvanometer. When either or both electrodes were placed close to the heart, no deflection was noted until the heart began to beat. During muscle movement conspicuous deflections were noted. These deflections, so far as could be detected by the naked eye, took place only during the contraction and relaxation of the organ', the patterns of deflection varying with the positions of the electrodes.

An important observation was that each heart beat was reflected on the galvanometer by deflections both above and below earth-zero potential and not by earth-negative potentials only, as was held by Lewis in his book, which represented the dogma of the day. 'Nowhere,' Craib later wrote, 'is any suggestion to be found that activity also gives rise to actual positivity in any earth-zero standard or context.'

He was, in fact, now challenging the generally accepted negativity hypothesis. 'Extrapolated to the normal human heart in the healthy body, during sleep or under an anaesthetic when most of the muscles are at rest, the negativity hypothesis, if valid, demands that during each heart beat current will flow from all parts of the body, in more or less direct lines, towards the lowered or negative potential brought about by activity of the heart. This would be shown if by placing one electrode on the precordium and the other on a leg, the electrocardiograph produces a series of monophasic curves only, indicating negativity at the precordium during each heart beat. But neither the laboratory heart in a spherical bowl of saline, nor yet the precordial lead in man under an anaesthetic or otherwise revealed any such radial lines of current flow; and it was decided without further ado, to abandon the negativity hypothesis as invalid and untenable. The true facts remained yet to be discovered.'

Craib then devised and carried out a number of experiments involving isolated strips of cardiac muscle enabled to beat in regular fashion. Strips were either suspended in air covered by a pellicle of fluid or immersed in a saline solution. From these he formulated a working hypothesis based upon dipoles or doublets which he specifically defined. The hypothesis not only conformed with accepted theoretical principles of electricity of what he described as the inanimate variety, but readily explained all patterns of deflection obtained from intact hearts and the cardiac muscle strips of the second set of experiments he had devised. He later wrote, 'In order to ensure that there were no obvious theoretical objections to the new concept of how cardiac muscle fibres might give rise to electrical currents, Dr R Canfield of the Department of Physics at the Johns Hopkins University was consulted. Dr Canfield generously gave his mind to the problem and agreed that in the context of cardiac action currents the term doublet might well be preferred to that of dipole.'

Thus was born Craib's doublet hypothesis.

Approval of his work first appeared to come at the Atlantic City meeting of the Clinical Association of America in May 1926. Craib used to call this the meeting of the Young Turks, since young scientists met here to read papers. In a discussion the author had with him in the twilight of his life, Craib recalled having told the meeting that his sole object was to present his experiments, adding, 'I'm not telling you anything, I'm not insisting on a point of view; I am merely showing you data which disprove the accepted theory. Please tell me where the method or my statements are wrong.' Nobody challenged his work. Walking along a verandah outside the conference room afterwards, Craib was accosted by a seated stranger who addressed him as follows:

> 'Look Craib! my name is Frank Wilson. I've just been listening to your paper. May I say that I am the unhappiest man in America today. You see, I know you are right and that I have missed the bus. I have been working for years on the very same problem. Like you, I have been most dissatisfied with the prevailing theories on muscle potentials as taught today. I have worked with Sir Thomas Lewis. I had just reached the point of conviction that what you refer to as the negativity hypothesis is false, and that currents around active muscle have points of entry and points of exit at the muscle surface. I've called these "sinks and sources" respectively. As I listened to you the full light dawned, and I feel it's kind of unfair that I should have got so close to the truth after years of thought, only to be robbed at the post by someone who seems to have done only one experiment in his life! May I congratulate you on an excellent piece of work. It has shed the glare of truth into what was hitherto an extremely dim corner of physiological philosophy.'

Unfortunately later on he and Frank Wilson appear to have been at cross-purposes, as will be seen. Wilson's dipole theory and Craib's doublet hypothesis became contenders for the honour of priority. Recording the above (remembered) conversation, with all the admitted unreliability of man's memory, seemed important to the author in his attempt to give justice to all who played a part in this account of Craib's life and times. The controversy will be dealt with later. However, it should be noted that in a letter to his parents dated 15 May 1926—a week after the Atlantic City meeting—Don wrote that he had met 'all the leading men in the country in medicine and was asked to present my work to the more important of them. They seemed to think it quite good and could find no flaw, so as far as this country is concerned, all's well for the new theory. So it remains to be seen what the heart men in England, Holland, etc, think at Stockholm . . . At Atlantic City I had several offers of what practically amounted to an assured career in this country if I'd stay on here for an indefinite number of years.'

But he was already having difficulty in choosing between pure research and clinical work and was bent on returning to London after his year's tenure of the fellowship at Johns Hopkins. 'A year in London', he wrote, 'will help to re-establish a perspective which has become perhaps a little warped by too easy a success here.'

Among the papers found in Craib's study after his death was a loose sheet on which was scribbled the names of his friends and contemporaries during 1925/26 for whom, he wrote, he had great admiration. They included Drs EP Carter, E Cowles Andrus, Perrin Long, WB Castle, Walter Bauer and Paul White. More than 50 years later he would speak of them and others like Dr George Burch, with warmth, for they had greatly influenced him. Perhaps, in turn, they admired his many qualities and the calibre of his thinking. Andrus was always 'Coke' to him; Castle was 'Bill'.

Perhaps surprising for so exacting a man, Craib missed the ship that was to take him back to England. The SS Carmania was due to sail at 12.10 a.m. on 7 July 1926, but Don mistook the time (ten minutes after midnight) for noon, only to find the quayside empty when he arrived to embark! But he was back in London in plenty of time for consultations with 'certain experts' about his paper for the Stockholm meeting of the World Physiological Congress, 3-6 August.

Generally held in the highest regard by the electrophysiologists of the day, Willem Einthoven was in the chair when Craib presented his paper. The outcome undoubtedly affected Craib's subsequent thinking about those in authority in medical science. Again he stated that he was presenting his data and his deductions to invite criticism of where either was untenable, for he was clearly challenging accepted concepts. But comment or discussion there was none, since Einthoven adjourned the meeting immediately after the paper. What was even more devastating to the young research worker, as Craib recalled in 1969 in one of his unpublished memoirs ('In Defence of Honour'), was being told by Einthoven after all the delegates had left the room that his results were at odds with fact and theory, suggesting, Craib thought, that he had falsified them. Craib did not stand mute. He apparently challenged Einthoven's alleged statements that 'everybody knows the truth . . . ' and ' . . . there's no point in further discussion', by posing his favourite question about gravity—fact or theory?, which he later also put to Lewis; and not being satisfied by Einthoven's answer that it was 'fact, of course' left him with the retort that there was no point in further discussion of his research because Einthoven was unable to look at it objectively.

Twelve years after writing the above in 'In Defence of Honour'—and only a year before he died—Craib was still deeply disturbed by this Stockholm episode, although he sometimes spoke about it in a jocular manner. As recorded on tapes at his home in Somerset East, he said that Einthoven 'told me exactly what he thought of me, my impertinence, my rudeness, but particularly the dreadful behaviour on my part to waste the time of world authorities on this subject and talk nonsense, heresy, rubbish'. Whether or not these recollections are accurate to the letter and, if not, perhaps unjust to Einthoven, they are Craib's perception of what happened, and as such must have wounded him deeply because he often recounted them in correspondence or in conversation in old age when scientific opinion about his research had turned in his favour. We do not know what later contacts Craib had with Einthoven but two extracts from a letter from the latter to Craib throw a somewhat different light on Einthoven's regard for Craib's work. The letter, written in English, came from the 'Physiologisch Laboratorium der Rijks-Universiteit te Leiden' and was dated November 12th, 1926, when Craib was working for Lewis in London. Couched in amicable terms, it was mainly concerned with slight differences Lewis and Einthoven had had about priority in publication of work on the excitation wave in cardiac muscle. One paragraph reads: 'Your remarkable work consists in the application of a very appropriate method; it corroborates and extends in an excellent way the work of Lewis and at the same time it supports my theory of the cardiac muscle segments constituting separate electrical units.' The other is Einthoven's way of ending his letter: 'How are you? I hope you will do your work in London with as much pleasure and as splendid success as you have done in Baltimore.' Craib obviously did not regard this as the olive branch. Perhaps he interpreted it as denying the originality of his research.

Before returning to London from Baltimore, Craib's intention had been to gain more experience in clinical medicine at Guy's Hospital. Instead he soon found himself working, once again as a researcher, under Sir Thomas Lewis in his clinical research unit at University College Hospital. On many occasions in after years, perhaps with tongue in cheek and in several closely similar versions (for he was a great raconteur), he would relate how he came to be associated with Lewis. He once wrote it down as follows:

> Lewis (on the telephone) . . . 'I've just been hearing about some experiments you've been doing in connection with the electrocardiogram. Would you come to my laboratory some time to show me what you've been up to?'
>
> 'Thank you very much, Sir Thomas, it is very kind of you to ask me. But I hope you won't mind if I say I'd rather not, for every authority to whom I show my work immediately becomes angry and I seem only to make enemies. So if you don't mind, Sir, I'd rather not.'
>
> 'I'm sorry you feel that way about my invitation. Anyway, think it over and let me know if you change your mind.'
>
> I considered the matter closed and returned to the wards and the autopsy chamber.
>
> A few weeks later I was called to the telephone again. Sir Thomas wished to know whether I'd have dinner at his home with

Lady Lewis and himself. This, of course, involved me in nothing, except in what was indeed a very great honour and an act of generosity on his part. So I accepted with pleasure and in due course was admitted into his very charming house in Frognal Lane, Hampstead, I think it was.

We had a delightful meal; my host and hostess couldn't have been more kind. I heard a lot about birdwatching, one of Sir Thomas's great interests, and met the family. I still felt myself to be very much a Colonial in these high up English homes, but having been in the British Army and in the 29th Division always helped in a measure to build up confidence. After dinner Sir Thomas and I repaired to the library—his 'den' as he called it—and sipped coffee and a liqueur of some kind.

'Well,' he said, 'so at last we've met and now you know I'm not such an ogre as you seemed to think that day I 'phoned. Perhaps you'll now tell me something of your research?'

'Sir, I think it is jolly decent of you to invite me to talk of my experiments. But, as you know, I've rather given up thinking about them. At any rate there doesn't seem to be a soul I can get hold of who doesn't resent everything I say. And I'd hate to make you my enemy too, especially after such a pleasant evening.'

Sir Thomas: 'Well, I don't think that will happen, so let's try ourselves out, shall we?'

(After a bit of a pause): 'All right, Sir, I'll tell you of my work at the Hopkins, but on condition that we first find out if words mean to you what they mean to me. In other words, would you mind answering a simple question or two and we'll soon know whether we can converse amicably or not?'

'Certainly! Put your questions.'

Craib (picking up a paper clip and letting it fall on the table): 'Please, Sir Thomas, would you mind telling me why, when I let go, that clip fell to the table?'

Sir Thomas: 'Certainly! The force of gravity, of course.'

'Now this force of gravity you talk of, is this a fact or a theory?'

'A fact of course. I'm glad your questions are so simple.'

Craib: 'You see, Sir, that's where the trouble begins. The force of gravity you speak of is *not* a fact, it is a theory or hypothesis put forward to explain all sorts of observed phenomena. But a fact—never! I can even put forward another theory. For example, that gremlins grab the clip and push it down the moment I let go!'

'Now you're talking nonsense, Craib. Of course gravity is a fact—all sane scientists know it to be a fact, and that gremlin stuff is just rubbish.'

'You see, Sir, I told you we'd get into trouble if we discussed what I call fundamentals. All three of the high up physiology authorities I have met say exactly what you say. You all seem to me to accept theory or hypothesis as fact in a dogmatic sort of way and teach dogma as fact. But my mind works quite differently. So I'm sure you'll agree to call it a day and at least we can still part friends.'

Sir Thomas: 'You mean you're not going to tell me of your work?'

'No, Sir! There would be no point. As you see, we don't speak the same language.'

'Well, Craib, I'm disappointed—very. Anyway, I hope you'll change your mind, for I'd like to know what you've been up to.'

So I returned to my lowly habitation in Southwark after an exceedingly enjoyable evening. Without question, Lewis was a lovely sort of chap whom one could not help liking and admiring enormously. Enquiries about him revealed, as I recall, that he came from a wealthy coalmine-owning family in Wales, with plenty of money so that he had soon been able to give up consultant practice in exchange for poorly paid clinical research. Laboratory investigations appealed to him far more than the highly paid drama and fame of professional work in Harley Street. As he once admitted to me, it was the empty chatter of wealthy ladies in the higher ranks of society and in their menopause, that eventually forced him to seek shelter in a laboratory, where the problems he studied, however baffling, at any rate never developed hot flushes and palpitations.

About two weeks later I was called to the telephone again.

Sir Thomas: 'Look here Craib, I've changed my mind about you, and I think I know what you're getting at. You're right about the force of gravity; it is a theory and not a fact. Won't you come and see me again here at my laboratory at University College Hospital and show me your work?'

'Well, Sir, if you really mean you can distinguish between hypothesis and fact, then I'll be delighted to bring my simple data to show you. But please understand one thing: I don't make claims of any kind. All I ask is for frank and informed criticism of the evidence I have accumulated which seems to me to disprove views you yourself appear to hold as dogmatic truth in your monograph on the mechanism and graphic registration of the heart beat.' LEWIS

Sir Thomas: 'Yes, I quite understand your attitude of mind. Can you see me tomorrow . . . ?'

Next day we had a long session, not so much on my experiments, but on the electrical properties of matter as I saw them, and about which Lewis had only the vaguest and most elementary of ideas. His physics was of the sort required to pass medical examinations and his mathematics pretty ordinary. My knowledge of physiology was of an even lower standard than his knowledge of electricity, but at least he treated me with courtesy and patience. He asked whether I had written up my work for publication, and when I

> said no, suggested that in spite of Einthoven's and Williams's* attitudes, I should now do so and let him see the manuscript in due course.

Shortly afterwards, Lewis invited Craib to work in his laboratory in the bioelectric field in a full-time post specially created for him under the aegis of the Medical Research Council. And so began his research career at University College Hospital and his close scientific relationship with Sir Thomas Lewis. So also began the watershed years of his life. The details of Craib's first conversations with Lewis, as he remembered them forty years later, have been recorded at length because they clearly show how forthright Craib could be in establishing his own intellectual stance, and how he would temper his handling of a potentially tense situation with courtesy and almost Puck-like humour: the gremlin**, for instance.

*HB Williams, eminent cardiologist in the 1920s.

**Of some interest in this study of Craib, perhaps, is his use of the word 'gremlin' in this recalled conversation. The Shorter Oxford English Dictionary (third edition, reprinted 1970) gives its origin as Royal Air Force slang, introduced in 1941 to mean 'a mischievous sprite imagined to frequent aeroplanes and to cause mishaps.' Craib must have meant 'goblin' ('a mischievous and ugly demon') which was certainly in use in 1926.

Chapter 5

Craib with Lewis at University College Hospital

Thomas Lewis was one of the outstanding medical scientists of the English-speaking world over several decades in the first half of this century. The son of a distinguished mining engineer and colliery owner, he received most of his school education at home outside Cardiff, found little in his studies to test him to the full and so spent long hours roaming the countryside and learning all he could about living creatures, especially birds. Perhaps this early consuming interest fostered a capacity for original observation and helped him to develop conspicuous manual dexterity.

Lewis started his university career in Cardiff and went to London for clinical training at University College Hospital where he was to spend most of his working life. In a recent editorial in the *British Heart Journal*, Howard Burchell (University of Minnesota) wrote that 'the young Lewis was early attracted toward a career in classical physiology, worked in the laboratory of EH Starling, and certainly believed in the scientific life exemplified by Starling . . . ' But he soon struck out in a different direction, embarking on what was to become 'a lifelong evangelic campaign to establish clinical science as a discipline, separate and definably different, from physiology and medical practice. In doing so, however, he repeatedly reaffirmed his respect and affection for these two traditional professions. His scientific and social independence probably presaged his lack of active participation in the great physiological congresses of the twenties, Edinburgh (1923), Stockholm (1926), and Boston (1929).'

It is just possible that this reference leaves an impression, not intended by Burchell, that Lewis was no clinician. This would be false. Indeed, his Department of Clinical Research combined the care of patients in the wards with scientific research in the laboratory. He regularly did rounds in the hospital and taught at the bedside, concentrating on the scientific background of his patients' ailments, which he used to plan rational patient care. For a clinician like the author, Lewis's book, *Diseases of the Heart*, is a gem and has a treasured place on his bookshelves. Decades before its time, it combines scientific method with clinical observation presented in language that conveys both the writer's clarity of thought and his clinical acumen. A few years after his death in 1945, Lewis's place in medical history was succinctly described in a review in *Clinical Science*, the journal he had done so much to establish.

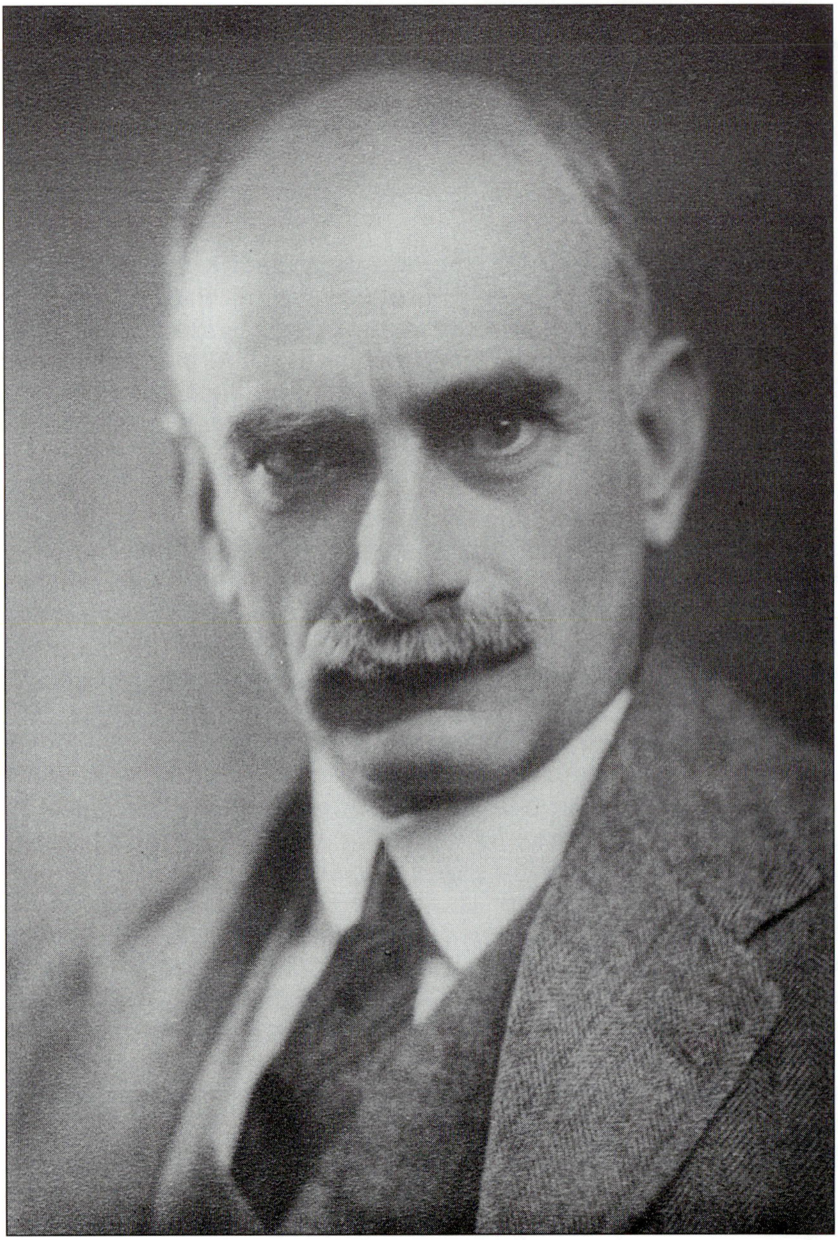

Sir Thomas Lewis.

'During his life', wrote Pickering, 'he had accomplished much; he had won international fame as a clinician and as a physiologist; his work had written new chapters in the mechanism of the heart beat, in the behaviour of blood vessels and in the mechanism of pain. What perhaps gave him most satisfaction at the end of his life was the knowledge that the cause to which he had unsparingly devoted his life was won; that the ideal of clinical science was inspiring men of ability; that opportunities for devoting a lifetime to its pursuit had been created and were likely to increase; and that the men whom he had inspired were united in a determination to further its end.' Lewis's scientific work appeared in some 230 papers in various journals, and in 12 books; and of the latter, Sir George Pickering, renowned for his own contributions to clinical research, regarded *The Mechanism and Graphic Registration of the Heart Beat*, *The Blood Vessels of the Skin and their Responses*, and *Pain* as the most complete and authoritative works to be found (1948).

Craib was just over 30 years old when he joined Lewis's clinical research unit. Lewis was at the height of his research activities and Craib was to remain with him for almost five years. Their social relationship seems to have been a happy one. Don liked the Lewises and in turn they apparently enjoyed his company. In 1986 I visited 'Clearburn' at Loudwater, near Rickmansworth, to meet Lady Lewis, over ninety years of age. She was being cared for by her daughter Pat and her husband, Sinclair Watson, in the family home to which the Lewises had moved in the early 1930s, shortly after Craib left London. Fortunately Lady Lewis's son Christopher was on a visit from Vancouver where he is in medical practice, and I am grateful to him and the Watsons for giving me a glimpse of what the home must have been like when Sir Thomas was alive, and what they remember of Don Craib.

'Clearburn' has a quiet dignity. Its aspect is across a valley. The house is surrounded by flower beds with sweeping lawns flowing down to a stream and dotted about with mature trees. At weekends, the family told me, Lewis's staff—housemen, registrars and research assistants—would come out from London to visit the Lewises and Sir Thomas would sometimes keep them busy planting trees. One or two jokingly complained that they did not mind the tasks given them but transplanting a young tree, moving it elsewhere shortly afterwards, and then transplanting it back to its original site later still did seem a little excessive! Today one can almost feel Sir Thomas's presence about the place. He was clearly never idle away from work. Apart from gardening, he would sometimes fish for trout in the stream; but his abiding interest was in the bird life. He was also clearly a very strong personality.

The home atmosphere must have been similar in Hampstead where Don Craib was a frequent visitor. Lady Lewis's one remaining memory of him was of a young man actively engaged in amusing her children. Dr Chris Lewis wrote that he knew she 'was involved with my father's and Don's disagreements and that Don came to her to try and straighten out their problem'. Unfortunately, Lady Lewis now has no other Craib recollection; but this evidence of his having sought her help points to the intimacy of his relationship

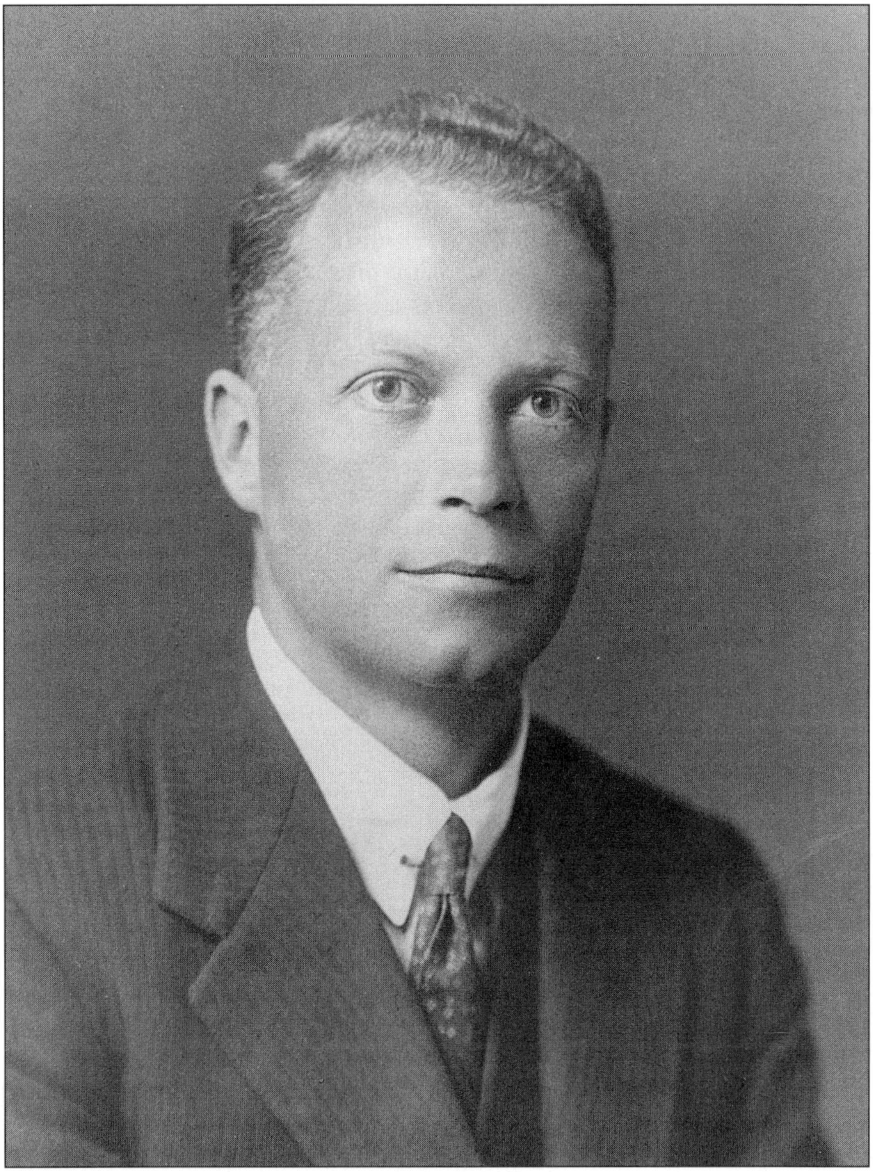

Don Craib in the Department of Clinical Research, University College Hospital, under Sir Thomas Lewis, 1926–1931.

with the Lewises. In the same letter (May 1986), Chris also recalled that Don Craib's visits to the Hampstead home led to 'anecdotes of his unusual acrobatic exploits . . . repeated over the years in conversation. I gather he was wont to stand by the fireplace and then place one foot up on the mantelpiece. He was also known to walk on his hands around the lawn for our entertainment.' Chris Lewis was a small boy at the time.

Craib's personal contacts with the family at home have been recorded to help understand his working relationship with Sir Thomas Lewis, their later disagreements, and the final severing of what must have been close personal and scientific ties. Some idea of what Lewis was like at work comes from Pickering's tribute, 'In Memoriam', which appeared in *Clinical Science* in 1948.

> 'Lewis was methodical and in his work a pattern was plain. First came the period of indecision lasting often for weeks during which he considered what he was going to do and how to set about it; he was moody and fretful and nothing was right; he would pace to and fro, appear in a room, stand silent for a few minutes with lowering brow, and pass on. Then, his mind made up, work began and, once begun, nothing was allowed to interrupt its progress, except his regular visits to the wards twice and to the outpatient department once a week. In his early years he worked extremely hard, all day and often into the night in the laboratory and then for the rest of the night and into the early morning at home analysing and recording results. Sundays and public holidays were grudged as time wasted. This went on for 10 months out of every 12. But for two months he was on holiday and then he would leave medicine entirely behind him and, no less intensely, observe and photograph birds. After his first coronary thrombosis in 1927 the pace slackened a little; he went home about five, and to bed by midnight, and he took up a slightly less exacting pastime, fishing, but the pattern remained the same. Relatively little of his work was wasted; for he was an accurate and penetrating observer and he made concise notes in his own hand on anything he saw that interested him, often laying them aside to be put together at a later date.'

Dr John Honour, who kindly discussed Craib and Lewis with me in 1984, was Lewis's laboratory technician during Craib's time there. He remembered Craib as 'a nice, bright, blue-eyed fellow; a marvellous chap—a friendly, generous, pleasant man'. He also recalled that Craib was working with the tortoise heart, using the most modern equipment available. Honour described this as a 4-valve DC amplifier with what was then known as a moving-iron galvanometer. An important point in relation to subsequent differences with Adrian at Cambridge was that the recording characteristics of Craib's apparatus were quite different from those of the capillary electrometer Adrian was using.

Lewis and Craib, Honour said, had much in common. Both were very clear thinkers; and they would be seen together in the laboratory having long conversations about research work planned or in progress. As described in the last chapter, Craib had been invited by Lewis to come to UCH to follow up the research he had done in Baltimore; and this he did. 'Lewis', he would say in old age, 'saved my life'. In regard to this remark, two things are clear. One is that Craib's perception of what happened at Stockholm, where Einthoven appeared to have doubted the veracity of his research work, had had a profoundly depressing effect on him (a common reaction in young research workers who believe they have achieved a major break-through). The other is that Craib admired Lewis enormously and thought he would be given a chance to prove the validity of his experiments.

He started working on skeletal muscle and soon found that his results coincided with his observations on isolated muscle fibres from the tortoise heart. Lewis certainly gave him every encouragement at this stage and the two men seemed to develop close empathy. With Lewis's approval, Craib set about the task of writing up his work. Incorporating his researches at Johns Hopkins, his first paper was accepted by one of the leading British medical journals and appeared under the title 'A study of the electrical field surrounding active heart muscle'. (Craib WH. *Heart* 1927: **14**, 71-109.)

Don Craib wrote another paper for the *Journal of Physiology*. The editor, ED Adrian, was a research fellow in physiology at Cambridge and an established worker in fields of research which overlapped those of the young Craib. Craib's memory of what happened, recounted many years later, was that Adrian wrote to Sir Thomas Lewis to the effect that the results submitted could not be verified and that he would not publish the paper. Lewis appears to have discussed this very amicably with Craib, who suggested that they challenge Adrian to a public demonstration 'at a neutral college' to resolve the discrepancy: Craib to perform the experimental work as reported in his paper; and Adrian to carry out his attempted verification. I do not imagine that Sir Thomas took this extraordinary suggestion seriously, but Craib's recollection is that when Lewis put it to Adrian he replied that the unknown Craib had nothing to lose if the demonstration came about, while Adrian had everything to lose. There is now no way to test the probability that this episode between Adrian, Lewis and Craib occurred in this manner. In the event, Adrian agreed to Craib's going to Cambridge to observe how Adrian performed his attempt at verifying Craib's experimental work, and such a meeting took place.

I have little doubt that Craib was courteous when he met Adrian. From his own account, however, he showed no humility. This should be no surprise from what has been written earlier in this book, especially about his war experiences, in which there was clear evidence of his having taken strongly independent and decisive action when he considered his thinking to have been correct. There was certainly no humility in his having asked a friend, who was working for Adrian at the time, to come with him to act as witness! Adrian, Craib maintained, set up the experiment and said it did not

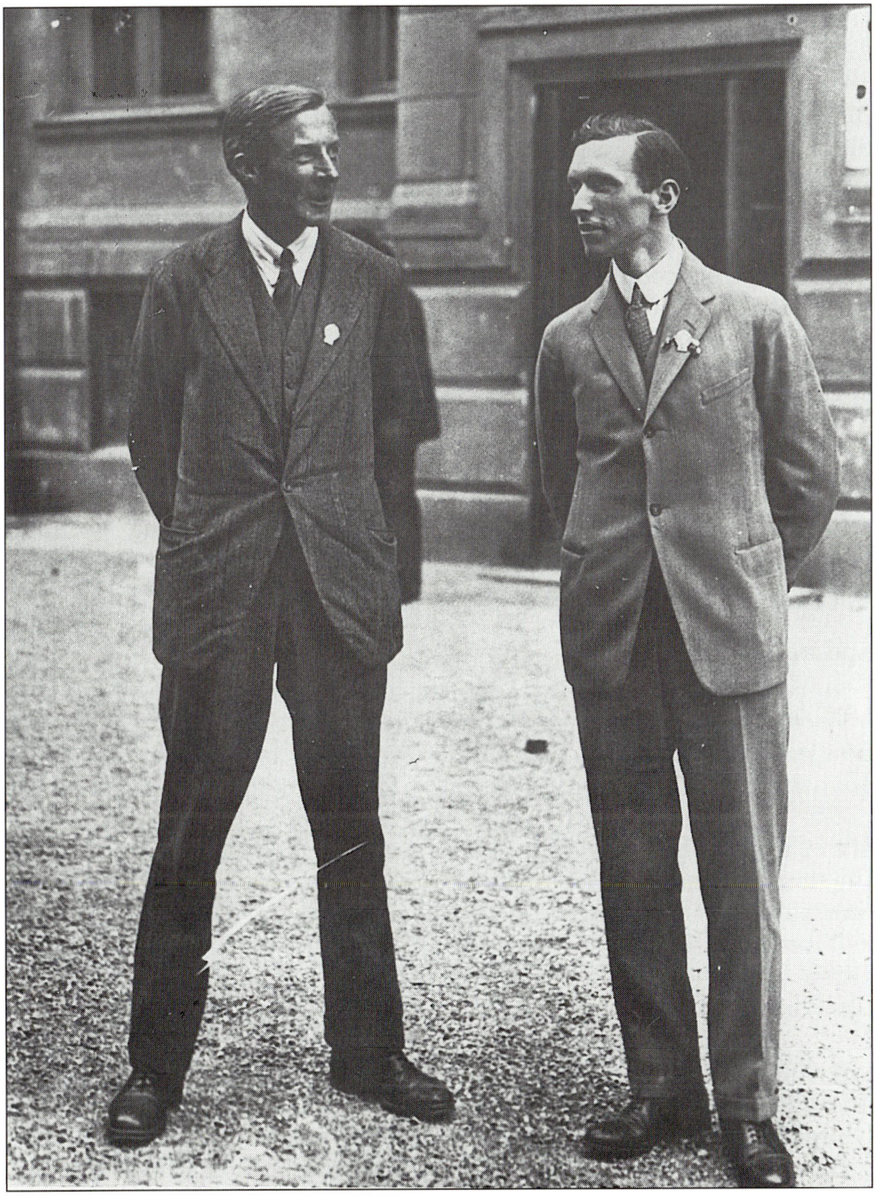

ED Adrian, later Lord Adrian, left, (with Yngve Zotherman) at the World Physiological Congress, Stockholm, 1926.

work, but Craib pointed out to him that the electrodes had been incorrectly placed, and not as described in the paper; and moved them for Adrian. Whereupon, the experiment reproduced Craib's results and Adrian (with little grace, Craib maintained) agreed to publish the paper. (WH Craib. 'A study of the electrical field surrounding skeletal muscle'. *Journal of Physiology* 1928: **66**, 49–73.)

This clash with Adrian clearly worried Craib for the rest of his life. He was to recall the episode in many conversations, and he wrote about it in personal letters and in unpublished memoranda; but he would not publish his version of the events during Adrian's lifetime.

Like Lewis, Edgar Douglas Adrian established for himself a very distinguished place in medical history. Born in 1889 (six years before Craib), he disliked his first names and was invariably known to his family and friends as Adrian. After his schooling at Westminster, he went up to Trinity College, Cambridge, taking five subjects instead of three in the natural-sciences tripos. His life-long commitment to research began early when, in 1911, he started working on nerve conduction in the Cambridge physiology laboratory, before he went up to London for his clinical studies at St Bartholomew's Hospital. (He was to qualify there in 1915). As an undergraduate he excelled at fencing and roof climbing—he is credited with having climbed a delicate twenty-foot spire on the roof of the hall at Trinity to bring down a white ensign, left there by naval cadets. During the First World War he worked on nerve injuries and shell shock in London at the National Hospital, Queen Square, and at a military hospital at Aldershot.

Back after the war as a Fellow at Trinity, Adrian started using new equipment for his research work, made possible by technical advances in valve amplification. As the *Lancet* put in his obituary notice almost sixty years later, he now set out 'on his great voyage of exploration to sample the activity of all the sense organs, to learn the code of their message, to see how motor nerves signal their commands to the muscles, and to learn something of the organisation achieved by the neural masses that lie between'. Recognition came early. He was elected FRS in 1923 and shared the Nobel Prize with Sherrington nine years later. The Order of Merit was to follow in 1942. Adrian succeeded Barcroft as head of the department of physiology in 1937; became President of the Royal Society in 1950; and later still, in succession, Master of Trinity College, Vice-Chancellor and then Chancellor of Cambridge University. There were many other honours from home and abroad, including a peerage. He was held in high regard as lecturer and after-dinner speaker; but despite these and many other commitments, certainly until he was aged seventy, he continued with his researches, often alone in his laboratory.

Such was the man with whom Don Craib crossed swords. Adrian's interests at the time may be judged from the titles of two of his books, *The Basis of Sensation* (1928), and *The Mechanism of Nervous Action* (1932). I do not believe that Craib's attitude towards Adrian was one of jealousy. In conversation, envy of Adrian's achievements never emerged. What is apparent, however, is that he regarded Adrian as one of 'the establishment', Adrian's background placing him in the British class which Craib so admired during the war; and despite Adrian's established place in what might be called the hierachy of medicine in Britain in the late 1920s, Craib would vehemently disagree with him if Craib considered he was right and Adrian wrong—a characteristic which is detectable throughout these pages. Craib had clearly demonstrated his bravery in battle. Justifiably proud of his wartime decorations, he rarely talked about them; but perhaps with episodes like this one with Adrian in mind, in old age he once spoke out as follows: 'I had been through a five-year war, I had won two Military Crosses for bravery on the field and a Mention in Despatches. I thought myself equal to any man so far as fear was concerned. I was frightened of no man on earth, after that war, so I could talk to all those Nobel Prize winners with the greatest freedom, without turning a hair, without falling over myself with respect, if you see what I mean'.

Craib worked for another year after the acceptance by Adrian of his paper for the *Journal of Physiology*, collecting experimental evidence concerning electrical fields surrounding isolated muscle, cardiac and skeletal. This basic research he later published in monograph form (WH Craib (1930): MRC Special Report Series, No 147. HM Stationery Office, London.)*, a key work for many others in this field and a model of clarity of experimental design and deduction. Lewis's previous work is acknowledged and criticism avoided. Craib's doublet hypothesis stood up to his own rigorous testing, explaining what was not explained by previous theories.

Although Craib did not criticise Sir Thomas in this publication, while doing this work he felt sure that his amassed evidence substantiated his belief that Lewis's book *The Mechanism and Graphic Registration of the Heart Beat* contained writing which Craib maintained was out of keeping with modern electrical theory. So he confronted Lewis. He would rewrite what he considered to be the faulty parts. We have no contemporary record of exactly what passed between the two men; nor, of course, are there clues regarding Craib's tact or otherwise in his approach and of Lewis's immediate reaction. Many decades later, Craib recalled being told that he was undermining the foundations of what, in 1981, Howard Burchell regarded as '*the* outstanding Lewis contribution . . . (which) will have a permanent place on the cardiologist's book shelf'. Craib's memory of Lewis's response was that he said, 'You have just offered to rewrite the scientific part, the electrical part of my bible, my book. Now, I want you to understand clearly one thing. I will not have anybody

*The electrocardiogram. An investigation of the principles underlying the interpretation of the electrical responses of muscle and nerve, with special reference to the electrocardiogram.

working to prove my book at fault. I have written the book, it's like a house, I've put on the roof and all that you are doing, and I cannot understand most of it, what you are doing is to nibble at the foundations. You must stop doing it.'

Craib, of course, had to accept this rebuff but for a time he continued his researches. He was, he said, studying vectocardiography, and proving that the human heart functioned just like the frog's heart 'or the heart of any animal you like'. But soon Lewis told him, he recalled, that 'there is considerable feeling about the kind of work you are doing, and I can no longer obtain financial support from the Medical Research Council for your work. Your work in the electrical field is now banned in this laboratory. If you want to go on working in this laboratory you've got to work on another subject.' Angina pectoris was suggested and accepted by Craib, who agreed to stop his electrobiological work.

Unfortunately Craib could not resist the temptation to continue with his original research. 'I became a cheat,' he would say. 'I used to go back at night and use the laboratory to carry on my experiments on the origins of electricity in the myocardium. I felt badly about it but I was terribly keen to prove myself right or wrong. I did not want to do anything in the world but to prove myself right or wrong; and then by day I spent the whole day working on angina.' John Honour remembers that Craib used to sleep in the laboratory and that he and other technicians would find him in the morning 'tucked up on one of those miserable examination couches . . . lying on his side, suit all creased'. Dr Honour also thought that Craib should have gone on with his electrophysiological research on heart muscle, because he was using sophisticated equipment (for the times) and was breaking into new areas. But Lewis got to hear of what Don Craib was doing and there was another confrontation at which Craib apologised for having done what he had promised not to do, and shortly afterwards wrote as follows:

'UCH
26.9.30

Dear Sir Thomas,

I think you must have been aware for some time that I have not been satisfied about my work here. The reason is simply that I feel that your department of clinical research is not really the place in which I can satisfactorily carry on my work on those electrocardiographic problems in which I am most interested and in which I can see work to do. I feel also that it is just from this point of view that my line of work has not met with your entire approval. We have often discussed what is and what is not a desirable problem to work at, and I have tried to bring my point of view into line with yours. I very much regret however that I am not able to do this satisfactorily. Since I can see no likelihood of my doing so in the future, there is no alternative to my seeking an outlet somewhere else.

I have not forgotten that when you offered me my present post, it was on the strict understanding that I should accept no post elsewhere for at least a year. I am accepting no post; I am resigning with a view to entering the practice of medicine in South Africa.

I also want to say that I am very sorry to have to take this step, and can never thank you enough for the kindness you have shewn me while working in your laboratory.

I have chosen to write this letter, for I should have great difficulty in saying what I want to say.

I am,
Yours sincerely,
WH Craib'

Lewis tried to dissuade him but eventually accepted his resignation. Besides Sir Thomas, there were many in Britain who clearly held Don Craib in the highest regard. Their views about his research potential must have been founded on his manifest clarity of mind and penetrating questioning and augmented by his striking presence and personal warmth. Several senior colleagues tried to persuade him to let his name go forward for posts in England, such as the chair of physiology at Bristol and a readership in medicine at Cambridge. But he again refused and declined to give his reasons. Late in life, however, he would say that he could not stay on in England because the people 'who controlled the money-bags dictated the research', implying that he would not be able to pursue his ambition to spend his working life in electrophysiological research. This view John Honour rejects from his own experience, maintaining that the Medical Research Council would have continued supporting Craib, away from UCH, had he chosen to remain in Britain.

Lewis reported the impending resignation to the Medical Research Council in a letter dated 4 October 1930. 'Dr Craib has resigned his post here', he wrote, 'and after going into the matter fully with him I have accepted his resignation. In my view it is a matter of very great regret that he has come to this decision as I have regarded him for some while as one of the most, if not *the* most promising candidate for a professorship of clinical medicine and research in this country within the space of a few years. Because I held that view about him I pressed his claims to full-time work in the Spring. I am now forced by circumstances to see that he will not work contentedly and in a subordinate post for a preliminary period in this country, and consequently his resignation becomes inevitable . . . ' The letter was completed by administrative details of no relevance here. In his brief reply a few days later, the acting Secretary of the Medical Research Council remarked that he was 'sure that the Council, when the matter is reported to them at their next meeting, will share your disappointment at the loss of Dr Craib'.

By this action, Don Craib cut his active involvement in medical research for more than thirty years.

Chapter 6

Craib at Wits

Don Craib spent fifteen years in Johannesburg as Professor of Medicine at the University of the Witwatersrand (1932-1947). When he went there the university was a young institution having its teething troubles; now, over fifty years later, it is highly regarded in the English-speaking world for its scholarship and its research achievements. Craib was to play a significant part in this transformation. Soon after his arrival, he developed a burning ambition to lift the medical school to world prominence from what he regarded as provincial mediocrity. But he was well ahead of his time and frequently frustrated. Nevertheless, with minimal staff to assist him and no research facilities, he stimulated students and his younger colleagues by his penetrating questions and his lucid thinking at the bedside, establishing himself as a dominant figure in South African clinical medicine. And he gave the university an insight into what it could become.

Both his coming and his going were surrounded by controversy.

Newly married, Don returned to Somerset East in 1931 with Doris, his wife, to see if they could live there, in his happy hunting grounds, surrounded by the Craibs and the Hofmeyrs who made up the family to which he was so attached. He would go into medical practice, but he recognised that for her adjustment in an alien environment might be difficult. 'The family tree of the Vevers of Yarkhill, Herefordshire, England,' he wrote later on, 'goes back, according to records in our possession, to the year 1603. Doris Eileen Vevers, born in Bristol in 1906, was a distinguished student at the Royal Academy of Music in London during the years following World War 1, and in due course was elected an associate . . . She still plays her 1695 Taningar 'cello divinely, and I have often been reduced to tears by the sheer delight of her performance . . . She has given me much that has made my life both joyous and interesting. My introduction, through her, to the world of music and ballet, and, in a measure, to the great biographies of present times, has added a richness to living that I would not otherwise have enjoyed.'

Their arrival at Gardiol does not seem to have been entirely happy, but more than fifty years later Doris remembers the meeting with those who were there to welcome them as a very happy occasion. It must have been joyous for Don since Gardiol meant so much to him; but surely he had mixed feelings about going into general practice when he had been so deeply immersed in medical research? Her first meeting with the family must have been an ordeal for Doris, as it is for most brides. The home language of the Craibs was English but several of the Hofmeyr uncles were predikants (ministers) in the Dutch Reformed Church and would use Afrikaans as their main language. Doris did not speak Afrikaans but the others all spoke English, so there was no problem on this score. Doris also recalls that she was ill with tonsilitis at the time and the hot-water system did not function at night, so she was unable to take a bath on the evening of their arrival. So this lovely young woman did not have the easiest introduction to Gardiol. All in all, as the days went by, it seemed a more sensible plan to abandon ideas of living in rural Somerset East and move to Johannesburg, and this they did: he to join Dr RL Girdwood in consultant practice, and she to take up her life once again in the world of music.

Before long in Johannesburg, Don found himself in demand as a consultant physician, and he was soon to combine what turned out to be a successful career in private practice with a demanding academic life. Doris resumed her musical career, becoming active as 'cellist with the symphony orchestra. Home life for the Craibs became crowded with their separate commitments, as they often are when both husband and wife have different careers and there are young children to care for. Nevertheless, Don clearly adored his wife at that time and his adoration was undimmed fifty years later. After the relative penury of his years of active research in Baltimore and London, he was able to provide for his wife and family in the manner he saw fit. And from a brief visit the author paid to their home in Saxonwold in 1945, it is clear they lived in comfort.

When the part-time Chair of Medicine at the University of the Witwatersrand was advertised shortly after his arrival in Johannesburg, Craib was evidently reluctant to apply. He had, he recalled later, already been passed over in favour of Dr Mary Gordon for a much more junior appointment, a registrar post. But on the last day, prompted by friends who recognised that his credentials were unique, like Harold Ramsbottom, who was an advocate and later became a judge, he lodged an application. The bare facts are that the selection committee, meeting on 25 August 1931, recommended the appointment of William Hofmeyr Craib; and Craib took up his duties four months later, on 1 January 1932.

Recording the events between these two dates in *Wits: The Early Years*, the historian Bruce Murray wrote that his appointment 'over the heads of a number of fancied Jewish candidates . . . provoked a major rumpus, leading to the resignation from the Department of Medicine of five prominent Jewish physicians'. This was a time in history when anti-semitism had reared its ugly head in Hitler's Germany, and Jewish people in South Africa, as elsewhere, felt threatened. Some may have thought Craib's appointment was on these grounds. Don told the author (in 1981) that he was summoned to the home of the Principal, Humphrey Raikes, on a Sunday afternoon early on in the affair, to be asked to withdraw his application. Raikes was apparently quite frank as regards the reason for his request: 'a section of the community which gives great support to the university will stop supporting the university' if Craib were appointed. For his part, Don recalled, he said he was willing to do this provided Raikes put his request in writing; which, it appears, he was not prepared to do. This seems to have been the beginning of considerable antipathy between these two men.

Then the Craibs were visited by an uncle by marriage from Basutoland (who was Director of Education there) and subsequently by the intellectually brilliant Jan Hendrik Hofmeyr, a distant cousin. Hofmeyr, one of the outstanding figures in South African political history, had been Principal of the University of the Witwatersrand while still in his twenties. He was now a senior cabinet minister. Both relatives came with identical pleas: Craib surely knew that he was unfitted for the appointment and should withdraw! Both requests were turned down, the latter with Don's rejoinder to his cousin that, as Minister of Education, Hofmeyr must know that he could refuse to ratify Craib's appointment, since he had the right of veto. 'You can just put a blue pencil through the whole thing when the application reaches you', were Craib's recollection of his own words: hardly appropriate handling of a cabinet minister but no doubt appropriate repartee between cousins! Craib was well aware that he enjoyed much support from prominent friends within the medical profession and outside it, and therefore let his application stand.

Complaints also came before the university's Senate and the Board of the Faculty of Medicine regarding the alleged unfairness of the appointment. No allegation of anti-semitism was raised. It was submitted that all four applicants—Drs Arthur Bloom, Loswel Braun, Henry Heiman and Craib—possessed similar professional qualifications but the other three were 'already members of the Hospital Staff and have served the University as clinical teachers for a number of years'. Craib, it was said, had no local standing and not much postgraduate clinical experience. The university did the proper thing. It set up an investigating committee comprising Principal Raikes, Professors Raymond Dart, JM Watt, Deighton Stammers, Ritchie Thompson and OK Williamson (the retiring Professor of Medicine), Dr AS Strachan (the venerated 'Archie' Strachan, the Professor of Pathology of a later generation), and the Medical Superintendent of the teaching hospital, Dr AH Louw. What was unique about Craib, they found, was his distinguished scientific background, and they saw no reason to upset the appointment. Perhaps it should be added that only two of this committee were clinicians. This is an important point if it is remembered that professors in the major clinical disciplines at the time (medicine, surgery, obstetrics and gynaecology) were usually appointed for their clinical acumen, their research abilities being regarded as less important.

The students, too, became embroiled in the controversy. Their concern and involvement was expressed by one of them, JH Gear (Jock) in a letter dated 4 November 1931 to his eldest brother HS (Harry) Gear in London. Telling him of Craib's appointment, Jock wrote, 'this . . . has given rise to tremendous heartburning and argument, and even yet trouble is brewing'. After mentioning allegations of anti-semitism and the belief that Craib was too young and inexperienced, he went on that '. . . it may all turn out amicably, but, as President of the Vacation Executive of the Students' Medical Society I am in a position to hear a lot about it. We . . . wrote to the Principal before the appointment asking reassurance in regard to the various rumours, e.g. closure of the Medical School, resignation of majority of the honorary staff, etc—that were floating about. The result was that the Principal informed us that there perhaps would be trouble, but one had to take a long view of the case.' And he went on to relate that soon they were informed that senior physicians in the hospital had already resigned or would shortly do so. 'I only hope', he continued, 'that it is all exaggeration; if not, to my mind, I see strong seas ahead, and (possibly) closing down the Medical School! It seems incredible.' A prominent surgeon 'was overheard by one of us to say that the appointment of Craib is positively ridiculous. So we hardly know what to think. However, that is the position as the students know it, and interesting, perhaps calamitous developments are expected. Apart from the anti-semitism which is alleged, the Selection Committee are looking at the matter from the academic point of view, and it seems quite reasonable to appoint a brilliant young man (Craib is 36) to the Chair, and I feel certain he will make a far more imposing professor now, and in a few years how much more so, than . . . ', concluding his letter with the names of several of the other candidates.

So began the association which developed into a life-long friendship between Jock Gear and Don Craib: Jock to admire the brilliance of the man, Don to value Jock's analytical mind, his excellence as a clinician and student teacher, and his loyalty. So also are introduced to this account of the life and times of WH Craib two of the three Gear brothers, known affectionately to many who came after them at the Medical School of the University of the Witwatersrand as 'Top', 'Middle' and 'Low' Gear. James (JHS) the middle brother, like Harry and Jock, was also to become a close friend of Don Craib's. All three Gears carved out for themselves distinguished careers in different fields of medicine and will often appear in the pages that follow.

The resignation threat was in fact carried out, RL Girdwood remaining as the only senior consultant physician. Five members of the Department of Medicine left, IJ Block and Mary Gordon joining the three unsuccessful candidates. The only Jewish member of the department's staff not to do so was IJ Balkin. The new Professor of Medicine immediately recognised the proportions of the crisis these resignations had precipitated. He could not see how he, Girdwood and Balkin alone could attend to the pressing needs of their patients in the medical wards of the hospital and adequately teach clinical medicine to their students. All his life Don was at his best with young people, and generally they reciprocated his interest in their welfare and his warmth. In the present crisis, he was deeply disturbed lest the medical students suffer. 'There is only one thing to do,' he told RL Girdwood, 'I'm now going to resign the Chair so that all those other people can go back and the medical students (will) be properly looked after.' But Girdwood would not hear of it; Craib must think up a contingency plan. The new professor therefore asked the Principal for permission to appoint (presumably temporarily) several physicians practising as consultants in the town, who were not Jewish. Realising, no doubt, that this would aggravate the breach and highlight the allegations of anti-semitism, Raikes and others persuaded those who had resigned to return to their work as consultants and clinical teachers. To help heal the wounds, the University gave a dinner party for the various participants—perhaps antagonists would be a better word—in this unhappy affair; and a genial atmosphere was immediately established by the bluff warmth of 'Breb' (IW Brebner), the much-loved Professor of Surgery who had that happy knack of being able to say almost anything without causing offence. At the beginning of the dinner, Craib recalled, finding himself seated next to Maxie Greenberg, Brebner said 'I'm damned if I'm sitting next to that flat-footed Peruvian! I want another seat', and there was laughter all round, the initial tensions dissipated.

Although some feeling may have lingered for years, this great controversy was ended. There is no denying, however, that anti-semitism was rife in the South Africa of the 1930s. In his perceptive biography of Hofmeyr, Alan Paton reminds us that 'South Africa was an ugly place for Jews at this time. It had once seemed a haven in a cruel world, but now one could not be so sure . . . Jewish parents were afraid that their growing sons and daughters would read the papers and learn that the centuries-old enemy of Jewish peace was not confined to Germany, but was now, in the words of the Book of Job, going to and fro in the earth.' (He was writing of Hofmeyr's championship of the voiceless and his active opposition, in 1936, as Minister of the Interior, to pressure for the restriction of Jewish immigration.) And even in the early 1940s when the author was a medical student in Johannesburg, anti-semitism was regrettably still alive, although much mollified by the stories of atrocities against the Jews in Occupied Europe. It must be emphasised, however, that Don Craib harboured no such feelings. In fact, Don had many Jewish friends; and later on he was to describe Maxie Greenberg, the butt of Brebner's jest, as 'a marvellous chap, a great friend of ours'. Embroiled as Craib was in the controversy surrounding his appointment, it might have been thought that he was a party to the anti-semitic movement that existed in the country—but he was in a sense the shuttlecock in the affair, not the cause. It is also important to stress that Bruce Murray examined the official records of Council, Senate and Board of the Faculty of Medicine of the University and found no evidence whatever that such improper criteria as anti-semitism ever played a part in its policy decisions or appointments.

As the years went by, old wounds related to the controversies surrounding his appointment healed. Two of the unsuccessful contenders for the chair he now held became quite friendly, he recalled; others who were arraigned against him later became close friends. Craib matured into an outstanding consultant physician; but what satisfaction this might have given must have been offset by frustration in his academic life. He was a part-time professor and was unable to engage in research. Nevertheless, despite the limits in time imposed by private practice, he became a great teacher of clinical medicine.

Craib seldom gave lectures. He taught at the bedside and it was there that he so impressed his students. He was much against what he described as the Scottish system of didactic teaching and although he was to tell the author that he always adhered to the orthodox view as far as student-teaching was concerned, it was quite clear to those of us whom he taught that he could not suppress his challenging habit of mind. Indeed, considering his record in Baltimore and in London, it would have been surprising if he had. Some of his teaching was certainly not orthodox: his views on diabetes, for instance. For the student this was both refreshing and rewarding. It was refreshing because much didactic teaching came from the other senior physicians; and it was rewarding because, for some at least, it changed their mode of thinking and developed in them a life-long habit of challenging accepted medical beliefs. What is more, many of us learned to look in a very critical way at the evidence regarding a patient's illness as it unfolded—the history of symptoms, the findings on examination, all the special investigations as they came through, X-rays, biochemistry and so on, and whether the subsequent course of events matched the probable course which might be expected from the diagnosis which had been made. This, of course, is, or should be, standard bedside teaching practice; but all too often the element of self-criticism is submerged under the satisfaction which comes from making a diagnosis. In the interest of the patient, a medical practitioner's self-critical approach is paramount. 'Could I be wrong?' is a very proper question to ask.

Craib achieved this by his own life-long habit of looking at everything critically. At the bedside students would be questioned—

almost exhaustively—about fundamentals. The meanings of words, whether medical or not, were constantly under scrutiny; and the validity of textbook dogma was often challenged. Not long after he took up his appointment, his students were being exhorted to verify statements they had made about their patients' illnesses by searching the latest medical literature and attempting critically to assess whether the accepted dogmas could stand. The medical school library, where, as Craib put it, 'nobody went before', was suddenly overcrowded with students trying to 'catch out' their new Professor of Medicine. If a student proved his point of view was the correct one, as judged by the latest scientific evidence available in the medical journals, he would receive a Craibian shilling. If Craib's claim was right, the student's challenge would cost him a golf ball!

And before long he was in trouble with some of his colleagues. Craib would teach that because so-and-so had made a statement or carried out a certain line of treatment, this did not necessarily make it correct. He was encouraging what he would regard as not only healthy criticism but also a proper state of mind for a medical student and the practitioner he would eventually become. Students began arguing with their clinical teachers all over the hospital in a way that was novel at the time in many English-speaking medical schools outside the United States. It was certainly almost unheard of at the medical school of the University of the Witwatersrand. One student, Craib recalled, challenged a senior surgeon regarding a particular operation he had recently performed. 'Why', asked the student, 'do you do the operation this way, when the *Journal of the American Medical Association* has just reported on 120 operations of that kind compared with 120 operations of another kind—and the mortality rate of the one was about 15% and the other about 50%; and you have just done the 50% mortality-rate operation? Why don't you do the other one?' The surgeon was furious. 'Who put you up to the idea that you must come and tell us surgeons what you read in the medical literature?', he retorted. To which the student replied, 'Craib said we must never believe a word he says although he is Professor of Medicine, until we have proved it for ourselves; he says we must go and read journals in the library.' It was the Craib of his fellowship days at Johns Hopkins now encouraging others to challenge accepted beliefs, and this was perhaps his major contribution as a teacher of medicine.

In those days of understaffing of the Johannesburg General Hospital, the number of students on each medical firm was relatively high. There might be fifteen or twenty at each ward teaching session. Craib's ward rounds were very popular indeed when the author was a clinical student; twice this number, or more, might attend, half of them gatecrashers from other firms. Many will still retain vivid memories of this handsome, dapper man at work as a bedside teacher, with a crowded half circle of students about him and his patient. Not a tall man but of commanding presence, he was never overbearing, and he never unduly raised his voice or used sarcasm to an extent that would be hurtful. One of his friends, WG McNeill, reminded the author of Craib's habit of pointing to a student whom he wished to question with the chest-piece of his stethoscope. And the student would know that the question coming was bound to be a searching one.

He often ragged his students about non-medical matters and delightful anecdotes about what he had said were bandied about the canteen and the common rooms, no doubt being embellished with the telling. Most of them were harmless bits of nonsense, but students liked them and kept repeating them. One that comes to mind relates how he confronted his own house-physician in the corridor outside the ward, took him by a coat-button and asked 'Who are you?', to which the young man replied, with admirable speed, 'Skapinker; who are you?': repartee Craib would have loved. And there was another tale relating how he and Brebner, close friends, had an argument after a game of tennis about which of their cars was the more powerful. This they put to the test by arranging them front bumper to front bumper, each attempting to push the other's car much like two rugby players would try out their scrummaging prowess during rugby practice! As far as the author could judge when Craib told him of the contest, the match ended in hearty laughter and no victory on either side; no doubt with much engine noise and shrieking of tyres. As Dr PJ ('Boet') Kloppers, a distinguished student who later joined his staff, said, Don Craib was essentially a fun-man besides the serious side to his nature. Those of us who later became his friends continued to be delighted by the fun which permeated his conversation. It shone through whatever was being discussed, helping to maintain a balance. This would sometimes surface on formal public occasions, as it did when Don, now in his seventies, was giving the address after a graduation ceremony of the South African College of Medicine. On this occasion, in the Great Hall at Wits, he first told of his visit in the morning to Professor Brebner who was lying ill in bed at his home. As he entered the room, his question, 'What's the matter with you, Breb?' was answered by 'Ah! Don, it's my legs that are worrying me.' 'That's good news, Breb,' quipped Craib; 'when you and I were together at the Medical School it was always your head that was wrong!' And this light-hearted opening gambit was followed by a thought-provoking discourse on jargon and the importance of avoiding it in medical practice.

Most students remember Craib the teacher as a well-dressed man, and even in old age he was usually neatly attired, his face sun-tanned, its features strong. Not that the effects were discernible to those who did not know him before the episode, a serious car injury sustained on a country road while he was engaged on a distant visit for a medical consultation, had altered what must have been youthful good looks; but he remained a handsome man. Many of those whom he taught during the Second World War will have vivid memories of ward-rounds conducted by such a man, now, however, resplendent in colonel's uniform.

At the outbreak of war in 1939 he was clearly eager to serve as a combatant: an unlikely role since it was now 25 years since the young science graduate had left Cape Town on the start of an odyssey which, as we have seen, took him to German South-West Africa and to France, and which was to bring him such military distinction. He was now an experienced consultant physician and this time his involvement was understandably quite different.

'Once again', he wrote, 'I offered my services to the Artillery, my first love, but was gently but firmly turned down on grounds of age (44 years). A non-combatant niche in the framework of (the) South African war contribution seemed inevitable, and it was not long (before) Professor Innes Brebner of Surgery and I, his opposite number in Medicine, were appointed as Consultants in Surgery and Medicine respectively to the South African forces in the field.

'We very nearly succeeded in having ourselves posted "up North", as the Middle East used to be named, but General Smuts intervened and ruled that the Medical School could not be further denuded of senior staff, and that we part-time clinical professors should remain in the Union, our military service being confined to part-time duties with the rank of colonel . . .

'Our duties were mainly advisory, administrative, clinical consultant and humdrum to a degree. We did visit base hospitals in Egypt and Italy for very brief periods during the war, but the nearest I ever got to a bursting shell was along a mile-long stretch of road on the crest of a hillside above Castiglione in Italy, known by the name of "Dead Man's Mile" or some such term.

'There was little in our war service to be proud of, but we did at least work long hours of strenuous endeavour to keep the clinical teaching in our understaffed departments alive, if perhaps not of a particularly impressive standard. The students, however, as I have known all Wits medical students to be, were utterly magnificent. To tell the truth, they taught themselves; today a high percentage of those who graduated during the war years hold important positions in professional service or in medical science in this country and overseas.'

In 1942 he came closer to death than on the hillside above Castiglione. This time it was not due to enemy action. A Lockheed Lodestar aircraft in which he was travelling to the war zone in North Africa, caught fire and crash-landed. 'Looking out over the engine embedded under the cowling in the wing on my left,' he records, 'I noticed the metal covering beginning to blister and melt, and black smoke trailing behind. Attracting the attention of a passing orderly and mildly enquiring whether this sort of thing was usual, he departed with exceptional celerity, and a second later we were told not to worry, but as the plane was on fire, it might be wise to put on our safety belts. A few minutes later the pilot's cabin was also on fire and the remaining engine had stopped. The plane was now gliding under control of the automatic pilot on a rapidly descending course to mother earth, holding her arms open in approved fashion to welcome us on our somewhat unexpectedly abrupt arrival. In due course we skimmed over a mud-walled structure in a small hamlet and hit the deck in what must have been a spectacular shower of stone, dust (and) mowed down veld scrub . . . '

Fortunately the fuel tanks were nearly empty so the aircraft did not burst into flames. None of the occupants perished. The pilot was badly burned and Craib spent some days recovering in a sick bay or hospital of some sort, recalling that he had spent 'a long silent day thinking about cats with nine lives and wondering how they planned the tenth to make it really worth while!'

Anxious to complete the trip to Cairo as soon as possible since he had medical commitments there, and no transport aircraft being available for some time, be begged a lift in a fighter plane being ferried to Egypt. By chance he met Wing Commander Vevers of the Royal Air Force, a distant relation of his wife's, who made the arrangement. He was clearly shaken by the crash and uneasy at the prospect of a long flight 'as part of the baggage in the tail' of the plane he took to be a Kittyhawk. Having completed his assignment in Cairo he was 'returned to Johannesburg, not by hospital ship, but by the same unstable contraption'. Presumably, this aircraft was also a Lockheed Lodestar. 'Having eventually reached home in Saxonwold, my face adorned with oil and gastric juice, I spent several days in bed to get over the nausea.'

In his memoirs in relation to this episode he refers to his first experience of flying. This was over the Somme battlefields in 1917. He was invited by a friend in the Royal Flying Corps to fly as an observer in a two-seater slow flying aircraft working on artillery observation and trench photography. He remembered that 'at the time our fighting planes, SE5's and Bristol fighters, held mastery over the Hun in that area so there was not much danger, unless, as was unlikely, Richthoven's Circus should turn up. It was a lovely clear morning, but my only performance as an observer was, I regret, hardly a distinguished one. My stomach, so brave and controlled on the ground, once in the air lost all its manners and in most cowardly but dedicated fashion dumped all its contents, mainly a big breakfast of porridge, all over the cockpit furniture. It was a long time before I dared show my face again in that squadron during an afternoon off. Sadly my friend Wyllie was killed by a German fighter pilot not long afterwards.'

Modern professors of medicine travel widely to congresses and other meetings, and Craib's disability might have proved most inconvenient. Fortunately, however, he evidently overcame his airsickness in later years, for he was able 'to journey by Boeing without clinging to either the seat or the air hostess! But as soon as the seat belt has been adjusted, I still feel very much like a full term foetus, warm and cosy and unconcerned, floating in the ambient ether, wondering whether delivery will be less eventful than that in the Sudan some years ago.'

In keeping with his fearlessness when he had decided on a line of action he believed to be the correct one, often on a matter of principle, Craib had several clashes with authority while in the army, despite his senior rank. The first of these was with General Smuts, then Prime Minister, who had summoned him. A large, empty ward at Groote Schuur Hospital had been offered by the University of Cape Town for use by army doctors for treating military personnel, on condition that medical students be allowed to examine them as part of their training. Craib objected strongly to citizen force volunteers being used for teaching purposes, claiming that these soldiers deserved the same privileges as private patients. He won his point after a brisk encounter.

He had what he described as a bitter quarrel with the Ministry of Pensions over the mechanism of granting disability grants or pensions, clashing with 'that intellectual giant Hofmeyr . . . a sort of distant cousin of mine'. He also had another confrontation with the Prime Minister. Craib had been asked for a consultant opinion on a high-ranking army officer, the hope being expressed that he would 'find sufficient disability to justify transfer of the officer in question to a less responsible position in the field'. The idea, Craib discovered, was to effect the transfer without loss of face. Full examination and searching tests failed to reveal significant disability, so in his report Craib certified him fit for service anywhere. Smuts again sent for him. In an anecdotal style which is discernible throughout his writings, Craib recalls the interview in this way:

> Smuts: 'Ah, yes, Craib, as I recall a rather difficult person. I've sent for you to discuss a certain medical report you recently sent in on . . . . There it is on my table. Do you recall the case?'
>
> Craib: 'Yes, sir, I do. Very well.'
>
> Smuts: 'Now, Craib, didn't you realise that what was really in our minds in asking for a special report from you was in fact a very kindly intention towards . . . ? You see, it has unfortunately been found that he is not really suited to the work of the high position he now occupies. We want to remove him to some less important position without any (hint) of personality defect on his part. When we heard that he had hurt a leg in a fall, we hoped to find an excellent physical excuse to transfer him with honour from an

exacting to a less strenuous task. You do understand, don't you, that your report has failed to help us to take what is really a kindly step on our part? Can you perhaps not change the wording of your report in such a way as to help me or rather help us to help him?'

Craib: 'Sir, I now find myself in a most awkward position. In the first place I cannot change a report that reflects the facts as I found them. In the second place it almost looks as if I am now being asked to help the higher Army Command to rectify a mistake in its personality assessment made when . . . was promoted to a post he was soon found to be unqualified to fill. I can well appreciate and honour the kindliness of the thought that seeks to rectify a military impasse without hurt to a high ranking officer. But honestly, sir, I cannot see that a medical certificate that has been specially slanted is the right course to take.'

Smuts: 'Then you refuse to do as we ask?'

Craib: 'I am afraid, sir, that that is so. And I apologise sincerely for not being able to help.'

Smuts: 'Well, Craib, good afternoon. It seems you persist in being a very difficult chap.'

The transfer, Craib wrote, 'was made in due course, but not on medical grounds. There are other ways and means of rectifying a military weakness without overt loss of face to anyone. In fairness to General Smuts I must add that not for one moment do I believe that the idea to slant a medical certificate for army purposes originated in his mind. It was conceived in the mind of the high ranking officer who first broached the matter to me. He, I believe, gave Smuts to understand that "they" had thought of an easy way out of an almost insoluble impasse safely, honourably and without undue difficulty, by means of a medical report'.

Don Craib had a great capacity to enjoy what he was doing at the time and he probably relished the comradeship the army inevitably provided. He must also have gained professional satisfaction since he was much respected for his warm human understanding and his expertise as a consultant physician. The anecdotes quoted above meant much to him since he readily recalled them forty years later, and he told them in an amusing way.

Although he believed that he neglected his teaching during the war, when not away on military duties, Craib certainly impressed his clinical students. By 1942 he had several full-time assistants to help in the heavy load of teaching borne by his department, apart from a number of consultant physicians who had appointments to the hospital staff. Among his full-time staff were PJ Kloppers and S Lopis. 'Boet' Kloppers was an excellent teacher. He became the first Professor of Medicine at the newly-established medical school of the University of Pretoria, but soon resigned to establish himself as a much-respected consultant physician in private practice while retaining part-time links with Pretoria University. He and Don became life-long friends. 'Solly' Lopis, a physician with expertise in diabetes and other endocrine disorders and a meticulous tutor of generations of medical students, remained on the staff of the department of medicine in Johannesburg in one capacity or another until his death more than forty years later. Lopis's admiration for his chief fell little short of devotion. And there were other competent young teachers to help Craib.

But when Craib started in 1932, he and his senior colleagues were part-time and he had no full-time assistants to help him introduce the kind of ambitious teaching programme he had seen in operation in the United States. He regarded the medical school at Wits as providing mediocre training. Indeed, he complained, 'I could not teach them anything except what was in a current text-book, orthodox text-book, of medicine'; and there was little meaningful research being done. Early on Craib tried to get a full-time staff establishment to complement the work of the part-timers and start investigative work, but the University was unable to meet the most modest of his requests. Nor could he drum up support from his colleagues, he said. 'I could not get anybody interested in, let alone enthusiastic . . . (about) building a medical school south of the equator which would be unequalled, with all the ingredients on the spot.' By this he meant unrivalled 'wealth of clinical material', unfortunate terms teachers of clinical medicine often use when referring to abundance of sick people filling their hospital beds. He had immediately recognised the great potential advantages of medical training in South Africa. It had a diversity of people and a mixture of first-world and third-world medical problems. Craib clearly had a vision of creating the sort of institution of high international standing now found in South Africa, like the present-day medical school of the University of the Witwatersrand and its five teaching hospitals; and Groote Schuur, the Red Cross Children's Hospital and other hospitals associated with the medical school of the University of Cape Town. Today both train students to become highly competent medical practitioners and produce research work of outstanding quality. Their standing in the world of medical teaching and research is high. Now they are similar to the Johns Hopkins in Baltimore as Don knew it in 1926. In fact, they rank with the best in the English-speaking world. Particularly in regard to research work, the comparison between the Wits medical school of the 1930s and its present status is impressive—and impressive by any standards. Almost nothing was published by the department of medicine before the war years, when the annual average number of papers was one; by the 1980s the department's research output was very considerable, with over 80 research papers each year, half of them in leading international medical journals.

Most professional men and women associated with large institutions like hospitals and universities experience frustration from time to time. In Don Craib's case, it is difficult to assess the depths of his frustration when so many of his friends, like Boet Kloppers, remember with so much pleasure the lighter, fun-loving side of his nature. Most of what he expressed about his years at Wits comes from copies of numerous letters he had written to others, and from scribbled comments and unpublished memoranda found in his study after his death. He wrote much of this material after his retirement from the Council for Scientific and Industrial Research at the age of 73, when he was back at Gardiol and had time for contemplation and correspondence. In old age, he clearly mulled over various episodes in his career, like his disagreements with Einthoven, Adrian and Lewis, and the various battles of his days at Wits. In my opinion his writings show much frustration, although he never described the events as such. Indeed, in our discussions with him in 1981, he frequently ended the telling of one or other of these episodes by saying that he had had a good laugh about it, as much as to say that there the matter rested. But clearly it did not rest, for the same set of events which had ended to his apparent disadvantage reappear time and again in his letters and other writings. What also came through when he spoke to us about his career was his belief that he had failed to fulfill the high promise which he knew his exceptional intellect had offered him; he often said he had been a failure, concluding such denigration with a laugh.

We tried to draw him out about his lack of research while he was Professor of Medicine at Wits. When he was appointed he had recently left Lewis's Clinical Research Unit after five years of whole-time research in Baltimore and in London. He had said at the time that his ambition was to devote the rest of his life to electrobiological research. Why did he do none at Wits? We knew, of course, that his appointment was part-time and the salary, in his view, meagre, making it necessary for him to build up a private consulting practice in order to earn the sort of income he would need for his wife and family. But could he not have encouraged others on his staff to embark on clinical research? To this he replied that for the first few years he had no full-time clinical assistants and the university provided no funds for his own research. Nor, at the time in South Africa, were there bodies like the present Medical Research Council to which he could apply, and the large international pharmaceutical companies were not sponsoring research in the universities as they now do.

'Could you not have applied overseas', we asked, 'to America or to Britain, for grants?'

'No', he said. 'I am a very bad person for asking for money. I had no standing over there at that time; I was still a discredited research worker'.

Craib must have spoken frequently about the need for research in the clinical departments, but in the Medical School he found little sympathy. He soon discovered that none of his senior clinical colleagues at the Johannesburg Hospital had any interest in research. None, apparently, had received research training. Indeed, he told the author that the only person in the whole faculty with whom he could discuss research was Raymond Dart, who was Professor of Anatomy and an active researcher.

Like Craib, Dart had spent a year in the United States on a Rockefeller Fellowship. An Australian from the University of Sydney, Dart came to be Professor of Anatomy at Wits at the age of thirty and continued to occupy the chair with distinction for the next thirty-five years (1923-1958). He ran his department with authority and, as Dean of the Faculty of Medicine for eighteen years (1925-1943), he must also have been a dominant figure among his academic colleagues from other departments. Dart was a man of striking intellect and considerable investigative ability, much-loved by generations of medical students for his oratory and his distinctive style of humour. There was often a theatrical aura to

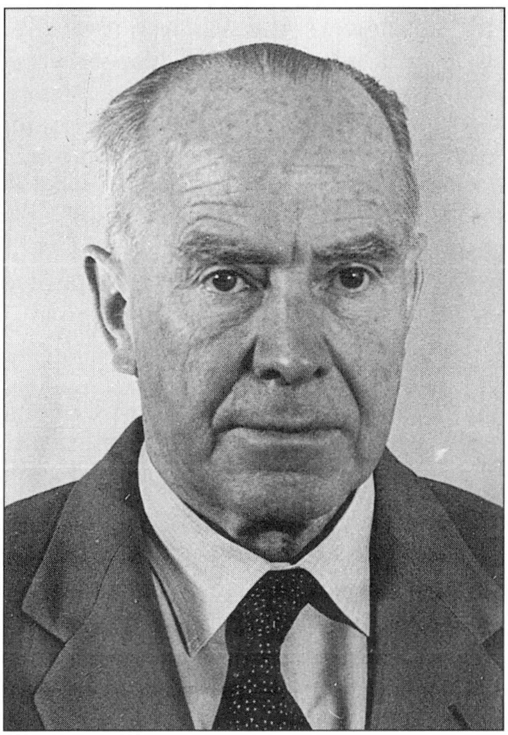

Raymond Dart, Professor of Anatomy (1923-1958), Dean of the Faculty of Medicine (1925-1943), University of the Witwatersrand. Anthropologist.

his delivery which students relished; but he was also feared by many facing their anatomy finals, for he was exacting in his demands of those whom he taught. He was, in a sense, the backbone of the school, a description he would like and so would his students, for his lectures on the evolution of the primitive vertebrates into homo sapiens were given with obvious verve, sometimes demonstrating with extraordinary agility how man became upstanding. He might, for instance, crawl like a crocodile on the long marble slab covering the bench in the anatomy lecture theatre to make a point: to the obvious delight of his young audience. And there were other antics employed for instruction as well as enjoyment. As Bruce Murray has aptly written, 'Dart's mind was an incredibly fertile one, full of ideas and suggestions, and he was never afraid to voice them, and work for them. He did not necessarily seek controversy, but he certainly provoked it, for many of his ideas challenged established norms . . . ' When he died in 1987, he was revered in the world of anthropologists for his distinguished scientific contributions, his well-deserved reputation stemming from his early work of discovery and interpretation of the australopithecine man-ape.

Such was the man we knew in the 1930s and 1940s. Such was the man whom Craib admired for his research ability and with whom he could talk about his academic and research ambitions for his department and indirectly for the medical school as a whole.

It is clear from what Don Craib wrote and from discussions with him that his early disagreements with Principal Raikes continued off and on throughout his fifteen years as Professor of Medicine at Wits. His first major attempt to obtain full-time assistance in his teaching programme concerned an appointment for JH Gear. Craib wanted him appointed lecturer in his department, with status as consultant physician in the teaching hospital. The university pleaded poverty but eventually Craib had his way and a post of lecturer was created which Jock Gear filled. Unfortunately Craib was not so successful in persuading his senior clinical colleagues and the hospital authorities to grant Gear consultant status. It is not clear why this should have been refused, but it is reasonable to assume that Craib's colleagues on the hospital staff feared an eventual preponderance of full timers, a situation which is now the rule in all South African teaching hospitals, as indeed it is in much of the English-speaking world. The hospital consultants, who, like Craib also had busy private practices, gave loyal service but had no time for research. With Johns Hopkins in mind, Craib's ambition was to correct this lack.

Although Don Craib had made a successful entry into private practice, he was apparently dissatisfied with his dual role as Professor of Medicine and academic head of the department of medicine on the one hand, and consultant physician on the other. 'I was very, very unhappy', he told us, 'at having to charge sick people fees at all, because the fees were going up and up; and by the time they reached me the patients would complain . . . ' that they were not sure they could pay his fee, having already been referred to several other practitioners. 'I found it very difficult to charge a fee at all to people in financial difficulty.' His acumen in diagnosis had become well-known. The pressures of his academic responsibilities and the demand for his services in private practice meant that his family saw less and less of him: a not uncommon occurrence among successful medical consultants. Most of them accept such disadvantages because of job-satisfaction and the financial rewards.

Don Craib, however, was frustrated, no matter how fascinated he might have been with the problems he encountered—and often solved—as a consultant. He had a vision of creating a medical school of the first rank, combining excellent tuition with high-calibre research. His relatively low salary as part-time professor made it impossible for him to cut down on consulting work to enable him to devote himself to his main ambition. He therefore applied for the post of Chief Medical Officer to the Mines Medical Benefit Society. He was appointed, he related, in preference to the prominent surgeon Lee MacGregor. 'A magnificent chap,' he said, 'a marvellous chap, he wrote a wonderful text-book on surgery . . . I liked the man immensely—he had brains, he had guts, he had character.' But despite this accolade, the two men had angry words on the hospital steps a few days after Don's appointment was announced. Craib remembered MacGregor's threat to report him to the Medical Council, apparently for accepting an appointment to a non-consultant post while practising as a registered specialist physician. Several of his friends warned him of impending trouble for infringing Medical Council rules. He believed he was in fact reported to the Council, for he wrote to the Registrar to the effect that he had not as yet asked for his name to be entered as a specialist physician (1938) and so had no case to answer. The Registrar of the South African Medical and Dental Council, however, has confirmed that no case against Craib was brought. The Register of Specialists was instituted that year but Craib's name was not yet on it.

More disagreements followed. Craib proceeded to have surgeons and physicians appointed on a part-time salaried basis to the Mines Benefit Society, but this apparently further angered the Medical Association. He recalled, 'They were absolutely furious about it and had a meeting about me.' At that time accepting such posts was regarded as unethical 'because a lot of doctors would lose benefit society money'. Like Dart, it would seem, Don Craib did not seek confrontation, but he often provoked it. He once told me that he 'did not have an enemy in the world'. It is hard to believe that this stemmed from naivety rather than generosity of spirit. Many others must have regarded him with enmity arising from the various confrontations recorded in these pages. But Craib would argue about a point or vigorously pursue a course of action while remaining calm and courteous, his mental agility and his logic enabling him to see quite clearly where a confrontation was taking him. There was no need for him to regard his opponents as enemies. Many of them would remain his friends—in his own perception; but it is dubious if all of them reciprocated such civilised behaviour. Throughout his life, as examples of this view of his character, he continued to hold dear the memory of men such as Major Maynard in South West Africa and Sir Thomas Lewis in London, with whom he had so vigorously clashed.

His salary from the Mines Benefit Society was three thousand pounds a year; almost three times higher than the remuneration he received from the university. He stayed with this organisation for a year and then resigned. The war followed soon afterwards.

Craib's feelings towards Humphrey Raikes, Principal of the University, must have come close to enmity, for they clashed many times. Craib would invoke a semantic argument about the word 'enmity' to deny this, but one of the entries about this word in the *Shorter Oxford English Dictionary* labels it as meaning 'a state of mutual hostility'. Craib and Raikes would fit this description. They had clashed over Don's appointment, frequently did so on the Council and Senate of the University, and clearly were mutually hostile over Craib's departure from his chair. Writing in 1979, Don Craib recorded the following:

> 'With the passage of the years, Minister Hofmeyr and Raikes loved each other less and less. Indeed, one of my most distinguished occasions was when Raikes, travelling to Fort Hare by train, and sharing a compartment or dining table with another Englishman, married to my mother's youngest sister, informed my uncle that there were two men in South Africa whom he classified as enemies numbers one and two, respectively. They were JH Hofmeyr, the Minister of Education, and Dr Craib, the Professor of Medicine at Wits; he named us in that order. Needless to say, I was delighted to be classified with Hoffie, no mean distinction at any time!'

Across the cover of a copy of the Adler Museum *Bulletin* in which this memoir appeared under the title 'For the amusements of old Wits Medicals' (1979:**5**,2), Don Craib had scribbled: 'Removal from Wits'. There is no better way of summing up his years as Professor of Medicine there and recording his version of his departure than quoting extensively from what he wrote.

> 'I loved the medical students at Wits. At first, they consisted of a mixture of white races only, but towards the end of my service there were blacks as well. By the time the latter were due for ward

experience and personal handling of men and women in hospital beds, social pressures became operative. As I recall, not only were black students restricted to black wards, but they were also confined to post-mortems on black cadavers alone . . .

'I can conceive of no group of medicals anywhere with a finer sense of priorities in a university environment, or a stronger sense of responsibility in the care of the sick in the hospital wards. Their manners, their sense of fun, their industry, their determination to understand before being convinced or committing to memory, their suspicion of properly motivated dogma, their impatience with shoddiness in the thinking, the reasoning or the teaching of their clinical instructors, all combined to bring about an atmosphere in the medical school that may have been equalled but which can certainly never have been bettered anywhere.

'This is praise indeed, but not lightly made. Having studied at Cambridge, Guy's Hospital, the Johns Hopkins Hospital, Baltimore, and having taught medicine at Guy's and University College Hospital in London; having examined in the finals at Harvard, Oxford, Cambridge, Cape Town and Pretoria, I submit that the assessment of Wits medicals offered above is not without merit. At any rate, what I have written is an opinion formed over the years of the many hundreds of young men and women whom I was privileged to know personally and to tutor during the formative, frustrating and not entirely unexciting final three years of bedside study.

'In the midst of his students a professor is at a disadvantage. It is not possible for him to know—really know—what his students think of him. But what Wits medicals did know about me, or rather what we knew about each other, was simply that as far as the science and truth of medicine are concerned, we were all in the soup together in an equal and equally humble sort of way. Authority and dogmas cut no ice; objective examination and honest assessment of a clinical predicament was all that mattered. For three years we were students together in search of truth about man, his mind and his body. If bluff there was, then bluff had to be called without respect of persons.

'Of course my way of teaching, with its insistence upon equality before the truth, was not without its repercussions. I recall one day being taken severely to task by a senior surgical member of the hospital teaching staff for inculcating into the students a deplorable attitude of disrespect towards their seniors . . . '

And he went on to relate the episode about operative mortality rates recorded earlier in this chapter.

'My personal frustration, if I may use so strong a word to describe a plight that never approached even the fringes of disaster or

> tragedy either for the school or for myself, lay in the fact that my appointment was a part-time and not a full-time one; on a salary, moreover, so pitifully small (£750–£1100 p.a.) that one's loyalty was forever fluctuating between God (knowledge, truth) on the one hand, and Mammon (hard cash and security) on the other. Johannesburg was then, and may still be, of the breed of commerce where personal success is measured by one's house, one's car, one's performance in society or the stock market. A silver spoon in one's mouth, placed there at birth, or by an advantageous flight of Cupid's little arrow, made all the difference to the path taken.'

He was clearly torn between the two halves of his professional life, but he vigorously campaigned for full-time chairs and the well-staffed clinical departments he hoped would follow. He had been outspoken on Senate and Council about uneven distribution of the university's financial resources, to the detriment of the medical school; and he pressed his case for the kind of medical school he had had in mind since his days at Johns Hopkins. 'I sermonised obsessively and incessantly in Council and Senate on the injustice done to the Medical School in a cacophonic crescendo upon every relevant occasion. No wonder it was not long before I received a hint too broad to be overlooked, and from Principal Raikes himself, that I might be better employed elsewhere.'

Mostly his pleas fell on deaf ears. He believed that it was on Council that he met the stiffest opposition to his ambitious plans, writing in his memoirs that 'it was here, I think, that I made myself most disliked. At any rate, Mr PM Anderson, Chairman, that fine and courteous man, was the only member who expressed any sympathy with my cause.' One day, he recalled, Anderson remarked about Don's relationship with Raikes while the two of them were leaving a Council meeting. 'You know, Craib', he said, 'one of our difficulties arises from the fact that what you say and what Mr Raikes says do not always tie up. And Council, for obvious reasons, has to rely on the Principal not only for information but also for (its) interpretation.'

'If full-time clinical professors were appointed there would soon follow not only a higher standard all round in clinical instruction and practical training, but also something hitherto lacking yet absolutely indispensible, namely, an atmosphere of enthusiastic clinical research and investigation. Wits had long ago established an enviable reputation in the preclinical sciences through publication of research of high merit and internationally recognised, but on the purely clinical side very little or no research of value had been published over the years.'

He must therefore have been delighted when a committee of the university's Council was set up during the war, apparently at governmental instigation, 'to investigate and report upon the desirability or otherwise of full-time chairs in the clinical departments'. In due course its report emerged, favouring the establishment of full-time chairs at £2500 per annum. But what he had always desired did not materialise until after the war. 'Indeed', he wrote, 'in 1946 it seemed that the impossible had happened and that a new era was about to dawn for the Medical School.' Perhaps he sensed that the new dispensation would pass him by. In the event, he was not to occupy the planned full-time chair of medicine; rather wistfully, it would appear to the author, he wrote in his 1979 memoir, 'The controversy over full-time versus part-time clinical professorial (staff) in a modern, high quality medical school was never settled in any definitive sort of way at Wits until near the end of my time in Johannesburg.'

'We clinical professors, Brebner, Black and myself, had all given evidence strongly in favour of full-time chairs. We had, moreover, emphasised that we were being forced into the degrading position of appearing publicly to support a part-time system in which in fact we had no faith. Had we resigned other part-timers would have been appointed in our place and the overall position would have remained unchanged. We hung on, therefore, in the hope that the situation would change, as indeed it did . . . '

When Raikes announced in Senate that the new recommendations about full-time chairs would be implemented, Craib rose to ask if the posts would be advertised. He appears to have felt that this was not necessary, and he and his two professorial colleagues were obviously upset by the answer that advertisement was necessary.

> 'Brebner, Black and I agreed that to be forced to reapply for the chairs we had held for so long was unthinkable. For me it was just another battle lost. We met in Professor Black's home one evening soon afterwards to discuss plans for the future in view of what was tantamount to the dismissal of all three of us simultaneously. We agreed that the only issue before us was how best we could serve the Medical School . . . I was fifty-one at the time, and by no means popular among the hierarchy at the University as had been made abundantly clear on a number of occasions.
>
> 'How well I recall that happy evening together and the laughs we had! We were really thrilled to think that the ineffectual part-time clinical chair system would soon be a thing of the past, and yet deeply saddened at the thought that none of the three of us would be there in person to see the new era in, or to help in laying some of its foundations.'
>
> ' . . . We agreed that to resign tamely, merely in order to avoid being seen as ignominiously dropped, would help no one. Something more positive was required. If the School were to enjoy fair, and not more than fair, handling by the Senate and Council,

the new full-time professors, or so we argued, should enjoy a status or power so impressive that they could or would not be as easily brushed aside as we three had been during the years of our ineffectual struggles to raise the standard of clinical teaching from our all-time low. But just how could this be done?

'In the end, after much discussion and with midnight approaching, we decided that the best way would be for all three of us to resign simultaneously on grounds of conscience. This simple-minded step we fondly imagined, behaving rather like the idealists we had always been in a hard, hard world, would invest our successors with the power to force the university authorities to play the game, not only towards the Medical School, but also towards the sick public. In true Kiplingese, which we had avidly absorbed during our teenage years, we felt that all the newly appointed full-timers would, with complete confidence, have to say would be: "Play the game, you cads, play the game, or we too will resign on grounds of conscience"; and the long sought monies would be forthcoming.'

Shortly afterwards, in October 1946, all three resigned at the same time 'on grounds of conscience', believing they were striking a blow for the school. It was probably a hollow gesture. Craib was convinced the university—meaning Mr Raikes—was determined to get rid of him so he did not apply for the full-time chair of medicine. Before the post was advertised, Don recalled, it was already being mooted that there was a strong candidate in Cape Town who would fill the chair with distinction. He was GA Elliott, who, Craib said, had a fine war record and had 'already created a great name for himself'; and in the event, it was Guy Elliott who succeeded him.

Chapter 7

Consultant Physician

Although it had been alleged that Don Craib was relatively inexperienced in clinical practice when appointed to the chair of medicine at the University of the Witwatersrand in 1931, this criticism was of no great consequence because before long it was obvious that his clinical acumen was outstanding. His opinion as consultant physician in Johannesburg, and beyond, was much sought after. He earned an enviable reputation and by the outbreak of hostilities in 1939 had built up a distinguished practice from rooms in the city. However, wartime commitments as medical consultant to the army and Professor of Medicine at the medical school meant the end of private work for the duration of the war.

When he resigned his chair and attempted to return to his old consulting rooms he found to his dismay that the promise that they would be kept for him after the war could not be honoured. The demand for professional accommodation was exceptionally high and eviction of the temporary occupant of what he regarded as his chambers was not legally possible. Elsewhere in Johannesburg the situation was, he said, quite hopeless. So he sold his imposing house in Saxonwold, one of the most sought-after suburbs, and the Craibs moved to Port Elizabeth, a large seaport in Cape Province. He used to say that he did this because rooms there were offered to him by a friend of his who was a radiologist; but surely it was also because Somerset East and Gardiol were not too far away?

Before long he was 'as busy as I could possibly be'. His reputation clearly helped. In his jocular way, however, he attributed the flood of patients to the fortuitous introduction of one of the first drugs designed to lower blood pressure. 'I soon found myself inundated with people who were complaining . . . that they couldn't live properly because they were giddy and were falling around and fainting.* So I had a jolly good high blood pressure practice, a subject about which I had a good many views.' But of course his practice was not confined to cardiovascular conditions. He was indeed consulted on the wide spectrum of medical disease, usually giving expert advice and bringing much understanding and comfort to his patients.

There can be little doubt that Don Craib had 'a good many views' about many aspects of his professional practice. Perhaps most notable of these was how he set about his consultations. The great majority of his patients were referred, each bringing a letter from the referring

*A side-effect of the drug used.

doctor. Not wishing to be biased in any way, his habit was to put the letter aside, reading it only when he had himself taken a full history from the patient and completed his examination. This must have been a time-consuming and exacting discipline but it was clearly in the best interests of the patient. Craib would first want to ascertain the facts of the illness in his own way without the intervention of the referring doctor's opinion. That could come later.

As many in his profession certainly do, Craib thought deeply about a number of the problems of medical practice: the doctor–patient relationship, the question of professional secrecy, the right of the patient to know about his illness, and the perplexing dilemma of how much and when a cancer sufferer should be told the truth (as the doctor perceived it) when the illness was likely to prove fatal. Craib would certainly not lie, but this is not the same thing as saying that he would paint the whole picture of the probable course the disease would take unless specifically requested. Patients have an uncanny way of knowing what they can handle and what they cannot, and this will usually determine their questions about a diagnosis of cancer.

Some of his correspondence and one of his unpublished (and incomplete) memoranda reveal his thoughts regarding this aspect of medical practice. The memorandum arose out of a court case in which a medical practitioner sued for substantial damages the surgeon whom she had consulted, because the truth about her disease (incurable cancer) had been withheld. Apparently she considered that in this way she had been denied second opinions and treatment unknown to the surgeon concerned. Craib jotted down his own thoughts about the several issues raised by the case, in the form of a question-and-answer memorandum, imagining that he had been called to give evidence. Asked by the judge in this imaginary court scene to give his views on the doctor–patient relationship, he replied at length. There can be no simple definition, he wrote, because there were so many differing circumstances. The relationship between the doctor and the inmate of a mental institution; a child; a badly injured patient in a street accident; an illiterate, uneducated person; a personal friend and colleague: all of these differed significantly from the relationship 'of a doctor freely selected by an intelligent and suspicious client'. And he went on as follows:

'I imagine that most of my colleagues as well as the public would agree with me if I were to define medical practitioners as a specially selected and specially skilled section of the public, and characterised by compassion and goodness and lengthy training, dedicated to the relief of suffering, and kept up to a high standard of ethical behaviour by the constant watchfulness of police and Medical Council.

'Where there is free choice of doctor, a man or woman in trouble goes and consults the doctor with confidence, trust and hope that his problem will be assessed with compassion, skill and care, that the advice he gets will be sincere and disinterested, and that if he accepts the advice a train of events will be set in motion that can only lead to the solution of his problem, the improvement of his health, or maybe even the cure of his disease.

'*The one result he does not envisage* is that he will be deliberately misled, that he has no right to the truth if he asks for it . . . ' Craib believed that the surgeon in this case had the right to withhold information, doing so in good faith and believing that this was in the patient's best interests. But he was adamant that the information denied the patient must be shared with a close relative or friend, an opportunity thus being given to seek other professional opinions or help from another source. 'The extent of the truth revealed to the sick', he wrote, 'should indeed be discretionary, but anything withheld from the patient should be shared with the patient's family group. The latter should always be in the full confidence of the doctor to help him share his responsibilities; and for free and frank discussion and mutual consultation.'

Don Craib was generous in spirit to at least one colleague. There were certainly others. Dr Geoffrey Dean came to Port Elizabeth to practise, like Craib, as consultant physician shortly after Don's arrival there. He recalls that he was soon offered consulting room accommodation by Craib and encouraged to embark on a clinical research project on porphyria, a few cases of which Craib had seen locally. Dean's subsequent distinguished research work in several fields owes much to Craib's support. 'Don influenced me in many ways,' he wrote to the author in 1987, 'not least in encouraging my research on the porphyrics, MS, lung cancer, etc. . . . There was no cant about Don.' Dean also took a courageous stand about a politically sensitive matter, to which he referred in the same letter about Craib. 'He stood by me when I was arrested by the Security Police following my letter to the SAMJ* about district surgeons having a duty to prevent ill treatment of prisoners.'

Don appears to have enjoyed his life-style in Port Elizabeth. Apart from the satisfactions of a consultant practice, he had a congenial home with whatever social and sporting ties he might want. He was sometimes consulted by national bodies for expert advice on medical education or research, but there was also time enough to indulge his interest in painting. He must be judged to have been successful with canvas and oils, some of his pictures being much admired. His talents were many.

Unfortunately, despite apparent good health, he developed ominous signs of serious disease for which the surgeon and a radiologist whom he consulted gave a poor prognosis. He was now in his mid-sixties and, as he put it, 'already returning fees to patients on whom I had made a wrong diagnosis. . . . It reached a stage when I could no longer accept fees with reasonable conscience.' So the

**South African Medical Journal.*

Craibs once again sold house, this time to return to Gardiol and see out whatever few months or years were left to Don. He accepted his fate: his father and grandfather had died from the same disease. He might as well enjoy life on the farm of his boyhood days and the origin of so much subsequent nostalgia. With time on his hands, there were so many interests he wished to pursue. And Don kept well, despite the gloomy outlook given him by his colleagues.

His colleagues appear to have been wrong about the diagnosis. More than twenty years remained for Don Craib and he was able to indulge his interests to the full. When he died, almost 87 years of age, the cause was an unrelated illness.

Chapter 8

Research Administrator

Don Craib had been living on his farm for three years, a busy professional life (as he thought) behind him, when he received an urgent request from the Council for Scientific and Industrial Research in Pretoria for help in regard to medical research. The Craibs were due to leave the next week on an overseas trip. With little hesitation, however, he cancelled these holiday plans and agreed to serve as Associate Medical Adviser to the President for three to six months. In the event, this appointment was extended, and later he became Vice-President of this large state-funded organisation. And so, for almost five years, aged 68–73 years, having returned eagerly to what was once his consuming drive to search for truth, he worked again in the field of medical research. These, he told the author, were the happiest days of his life.

After the Second World War, the government of General Smuts had established this council and appointed Dr Basil Schonland as its head. Schonland immediately appealed to Craib to become secretary for medical research, but Don declined. He had shared rooms with Basil Schonland at Cambridge and Basil had married his sister Ismay. 'I would like to serve under you,' he told his brother-in-law, 'but I cannot take (the post) because it would be an example of nepotism.' Perhaps he was to regret this commendable stand, taken on principle, because he soon became embroiled in the controversy at Wits regarding the creation of full-time chairs which led to his resignation as part-time Professor of Medicine.

After leaving the University of the Witwatersrand, Craib served on several government commissions, including the Du Toit Commission on Medical Research. For some years he advised the funding authority (the Department of National Education) on the budgetary submissions of the Faculty of Medicine of the University of Natal, paying frequent visits to the medical school in Durban. It was in this capacity that Craib renewed his contacts with the author, transforming the one-time professor-student relationship into a happy communion between colleagues and a lasting friendship (as he did with so many others). His services were sought by many national bodies because of his past experience and unchallenged standing in medical education and research—and his clear and detached approach to problems of any kind.

Many years of his life had been spent on medical research in Baltimore and in London. Indeed, at the time his ambition was to spend his life in electrophysiological research. He had abandoned

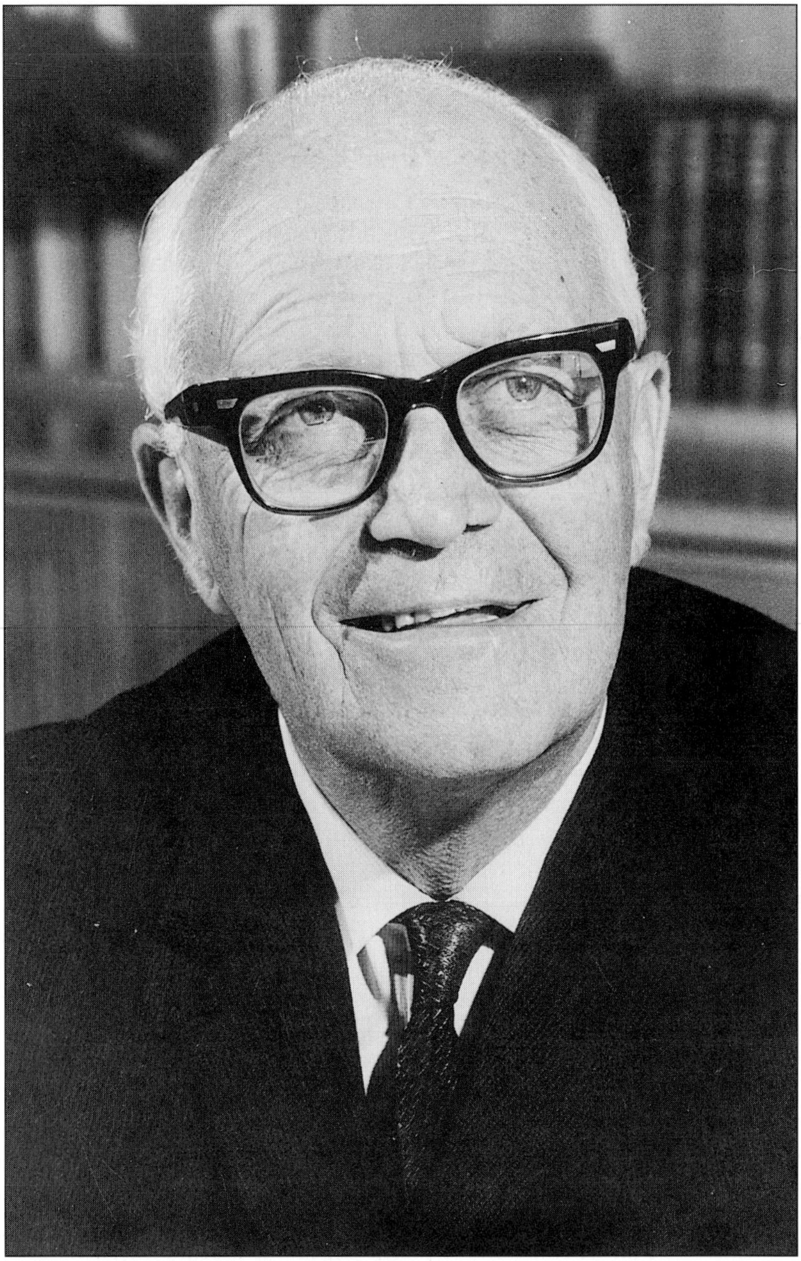

WH Craib, Vice-President, CSIR, Pretoria.

this part of his career largely because of his intense dissatisfaction with what he felt was unnecessarily tight control of what research may be undertaken and how it was funded. He had rebelled against the dominance of authority. So, although now far removed from active research and even from the practice of medicine, given the opportunity to influence the organisation of medical research in South Africa, Craib seems to have accepted with enthusiasm the offer which came to him so unexpectedly.

He was well-fitted for the tasks ahead.

In a scrap-book of his CSIR years (1963–68), Don composed one of his several soliloquies. Another will appear at the end of this book. In the margin was scribbled: 'Spirit of enquiry is (the) measure of a civilisation.' The editing is the author's. This perhaps should be regarded as the title of what followed.

'There is within man something that distinguishes him from animals', he wrote, 'and that is the quality that makes him ask why. Animals ask how, but man is concerned with both how and why and he cannot help himself. People differ from each other in their initiative and dedication to know how and why, and (in) a small percentage this persistence (in questioning) is developed to such heights (as) almost to be abnormal.

'To man, mystery is a dare to unmask; to the higher grades of man the dare is overwhelming, to the lower grades . . . the mystery is accepted in a defeatist kind of way, and becomes part of a mystical world attributed to deities, devils and spirits. Dedication to find out how and why becomes a hallmark of intelligence . . .

'In my experience in Britain 45 years ago, there was little control of research—and little guidance or direction. Research workers were regarded as odd bods, nonconforming mental and spiritual adventurers, rara avis types differing from their fellows, and looked down on rather than up to because they were spending their energies on things that carried no social advantage or advancement, no security, no material gain. Research was a sort of game played by individuals in a lonely sort of way. Research workers looked pale and untidy and did not play the proper manly games that normal people conventionally indulged in. Certainly Britain (Empire) had not yet entered the international rat race of medical research of today, and lagged far behind the Continent and the States in enthusiasm and financial resources.

'But a beginning had been made. Mackenzie, Lewis, Adrian, Haldane, Hopkins, Sherrington, Sharpey-Shaeffer, AV Hill were becoming established in an international sense—and by 1928 international pride in medical research achievement was recognised and becoming competitive. The race was on . . . ' And now the researcher in Craib wanted to make another contribution.

Administration, especially in a state-funded institution, is a difficult field in which to shine, but this is what Craib did. Not that his own administrative talents were particularly noteworthy. Fortunately in this he was ably assisted by that wise and astute administrator, Murray Baxter. Murray and Don became close friends whose critical approach to problems was mutually appealing. Craib would pose all manner of problems to Baxter, even after Craib's CSIR years, and the answers, some of which are extant, reveal how the debate went on between them.

What Don Craib achieved was an aura of scientific integrity and enquiry that was both essential for the development of medical research, and highly stimulating to active research workers, aspirant or renowned. His sense of humour, too, shone through in all his dealings with others, and he was much-loved for this. Nobody with an idea was trampled under. Every researcher, established or not, was given sympathetic hearing and enthusiastic encouragement to seek the truth no matter how this might run counter to currently held practice or belief. Dogma was an invitation to challenge.

Craib's area of activity in CSIR was coordinated in the Committee for Research in Medical Sciences on which the author served for a number of years. Usually to be seen quietly sitting next to the chairman, his own intervention in the debates coming only when invited, Craib's influence was considerable. Always a courteous man, he would invariably come to the core of a problem without circumlocution—an endearing quality in any committee with an extensive agenda. (Deliberations of this committee, meeting biennially, generally lasted two days). Most of the work involved grants for the various research units supported by CSIR as well as

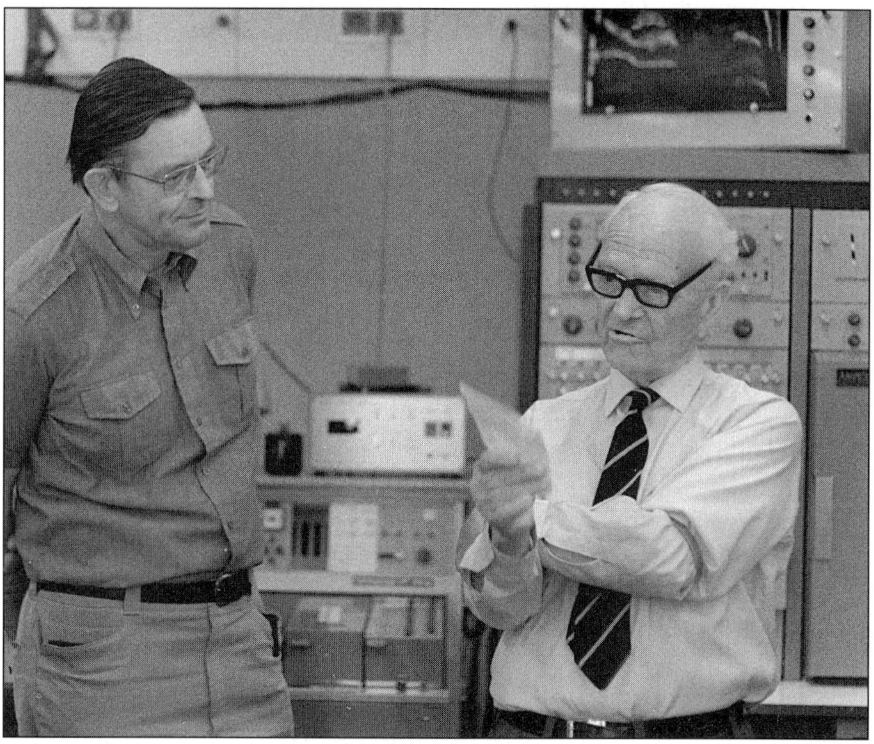

Craib as research administrator: nobody with an idea was brushed aside or hurriedly dealt with; much time was spent in asking questions, occasionally in giving advice.

for individual research workers. Don's activities included visits to the units and to lone researchers, and it was here that his influence was greatest. Nobody with an idea was brushed aside or hurriedly dealt with. He spent much time asking questions; occasionally he gave advice.

While he was at CSIR and afterwards, Craib tried to ensure that an electrical engineer of considerable ability, Karl Posel, was given a sympathetic hearing and adequate financial support in his attempts to apply engineering principles to the solution of a major medical problem—the management of the acute heart attack. Dr Posel, who was not medically qualified, tried to move medical thinking away from the coronary arteries as the root cause of the attack, directing research endeavour to energy imbalance. Craib felt that Posel, who had an original bio-engineering approach, deserved whatever support could be found for him and his collaborators, particularly Dr Ninian Lamont, a consultant physician on the staff of a major Durban hospital. It is clear from correspondence between both of them and Don Craib that they valued his encouragement and critical questions. Craib was instrumental in persuading the CSIR, the University of Natal and the Natal Provincial Administration to finance both Posel's basic work and the clinical appraisal which should stem from it. Posel was given a research fellowship in the University of Natal, and a clinical unit under Lamont was set up at Addington Hospital.

Don Craib's own frustrating experience as a research worker in the 1920s, his belief that there was much to be offered to the progress of clinical medicine by using engineering know-how (he often called himself an engineer turned physician), and his insistence on finding the truth about a problem no matter what opinions might be held, no doubt spurred him on to help this project. He and the author constituted a two-man committee to advise the funding bodies. The obstacles to be overcome were many. First there was the disbelief of the medical profession. Then there was the fact that only Posel understood the mathematical basis upon which his team relied when making clinical decisions on patients, but he was not legally entitled to give orders to the nursing staff. Many academic clinicians, the author included, were adamant that properly designed clinical trials were essential if claims about the efficacy of an almost revolutionary treatment regimen were to carry any conviction. And finally, no definition of what constituted a 'heart attack' which practising physicians could accept was forthcoming; and Craib himself could not be satisfied about definition of a number of terms used in the research reports. So the project finally lost both momentum and funding. In retrospect, what was so important about Craib's involvement was the way in which he doggedly persisted in his own support and criticism until he was satisfied that the researchers concerned had had ample opportunity to prove their point—without the heavy hand of authority unjustifiably crushing their efforts.

One of the fields of research with which Craib was involved as an administrator was bilharzia. The disease in man is caused by schistosomes (mostly *Schistosoma haematobium* in South Africa). To study it, the CSIR had established a research unit in the small town of Nelspruit, nestling among the mountains of the Eastern Transvaal. Here the disease is rife because there is considerable schistosomal infestation of the vector snail which inhabits the streams and rivers abounding in this area of great scenic beauty, relatively affluent farmers and poverty-stricken Africans. Many of the latter live in scattered villages and theirs is a subsistence economy. Educational standards, although improving, are still low. The children delight in bathing in the rivers, where they are infected by bilharzia.

The funding of bilharzia research posed problems for CSIR. Without doubt, there was a very high rate of infestation of African children in both Eastern Transvaal and Natal where the rivers flow into the Indian ocean. On the one hand, parasitologists and health administrators held strong views that the problem was of such proportions that heavy state funding was imperative. On the other, paediatricians and physicians were adamant that, curiously enough, the amount of morbidity (actual disease) seen in their hospital wards did not justify a high priority when it came to research funding, the research budget being limited. Craib was fully aware of this dichotomy of medical opinion and was most concerned, as administrator, to reach a balanced view. The problem is still not solved. Craib's papers leave no doubt that he thought deeply about the bigger (but related) problem of the funding of 'pure' versus applied research; perhaps he remembered his own views at the time he worked for Lewis and once again wrestled with the dilemma Lewis had faced over continuing to seek financial support from the Medical Research Council for Craib's fundamental research.

On one occasion at Nelspruit, where CSIR officials were meeting with others involved in bilharzia research, he was asked to make an after-dinner speech dealing with the opposing opinions expressed at the conference: not an easy task when feelings are high. With much fun-making and much good sense, he outlined the dilemma—to the amusement of his listeners and perhaps to their discomfort, for Craib faced both sides of the controversy with uncomfortable facts.

During this period, perhaps surprisingly, he actively contributed to the field of research on bilharzia by writing a thought-provoking scientific paper under the title 'Final resting place and egg-laying sites of bilharzial schistosomes in man in South Africa'. (*Central African Medical Journal*, 1968: **14**, 72.)

His sense of humour shone through in all his dealings with others, and he was much-loved for this.

Don Craib frequently mixed the serious side of his work with fun, sometimes invoking his sense of humour on the most unexpected occasion. At CSIR, most of his colleagues, in one way or another, experienced something of the fun he brought to life. Sometimes, but by no means always, his humour could be described as Puck-like. The first entry about Puck in the *Oxford Reference Dictionary* reads: 'A merry mischievous sprite or goblin'. The other entry, an older usage, is that Puck was an evil demon. The latter Craib was not, but most who knew him well (and some who did not), will remember his humour as certainly merry and often good-naturedly mischievous. Anecdotes abound. Three are worth quoting. For two of them I am indebted to Murray Baxter.

The first concerns his great friend, Dr PJ du Toit, a scientist of distinction and former director of the internationally renowned Institute of Veterinary Research at Onderstepoort, outside Pretoria in the Transvaal. Du Toit was one of a small band of South Africans who were elected FRS, and had been caretaker President of CSIR between two other remarkable men, Basil Schonland and Meiring Naude. Baxter described him as 'a smallish man with a large head and a very impressive presence; a man with a sonorous voice, full-bodied and rich, with an outstanding command of English and Afrikaans; a raconteur, a wit, an after-dinner speaker of distinction with an inexhaustible reservoir of jokes, and an obsession—almost—about numbers . . . He would see obscure relationships in the numbers on motorcar number plates. Sometimes, when travelling to meetings by car, he would challenge the other occupants to establish all the possible combinations on the number plates we were passing or following . . . ' Apart from 'his Onderstepoort achievements, his FRS and other national and international honours,' Baxter continues, 'he had an eye for a pretty woman'. Don perhaps did not have 'an eye' but was invariably charming. No wonder, intellectually and fun-wise, the two were friends. When Meiring Naude became President of CSIR, du Toit was retained as an adviser on biological matters.

Baxter's first anecdote is about 'a journey by car to a meeting in Johannesburg. I was in front with a driver and in the back there were Don Craib, PJ, and between them Jeanette Swanepoel, my committee clerk. It started right from the beginning. They vied for the attention of Jeanette. They flirted with her outrageously. They made the most scurrilous remarks about each other. Each took one of Jeanette's hands and held it all the way to Johannesburg. At one time PJ instructed the driver to stop, saying that Dr Craib wanted to get out of the car and hitch-hike. In fact for a moment the driver, startled, slowed down until I nudged him. Their verbal shafts aimed at each other ranged from the rapier wit of a Shaw or an Oscar Wilde to the "sticks and stones" type of ragging of a standard five schoolboy.

'I have an enduring memory of Jeanette, sitting bolt upright with both her hands captive, her cheeks flushed, her brown eyes sparkling as her glances darted from one to the other, not saying a word while these two duellists fought for her favours.

'Afterwards Jeanette told me that her nose tickled maddeningly but she dared not release one of her hands in case one of them would claim victory.'

In 1971, having been sent *In Defence of Honour*, Craib's light-hearted defence of his research record and his disagreements with Einthoven, Lewis and others in the 1920s, one of Don Craib's long-standing English friends wrote to another that ' . . . while Craib in one sense remains firmly on the ground, he is always capable of walking on his hands if he feels like it or the action seems appropriate'. Baxter's second anecdote bears this out. Unexpectedly asked to give the after-dinner speech at a function while engaged on one of his visits to an outlying bilharzia research unit funded by CSIR, Don caused great merriment and no doubt some amazement by miming throughout the time he was on his feet. Not a word was uttered, his changing facial expressions and his body language mimicking the sort of speech the diners expected.

Don was sometimes almost merciless in his ragging. From what he told us at Somerset East the year before his death, he often chaffed Afrikaans-speaking colleagues about their possible membership of the Broederbond. This organisation appears to have been an exclusive one, membership being tightly-controlled and limited to Afrikaners. It had no official standing but clearly exerted considerable influence on the running of the state, including the making of key appointments. English-speakers disliked it intensely and the English-language press was vehement in its condemnation of the extraparliamentary control it clearly exercised.

When sitting on a committee composed entirely of Afrikaners, Don would quip that he knew that most of them were 'Broeders' but could not say so, that they must understand that he was a b . . . Englishman (this despite his Scottish-Afrikaner ancestry) and that if they had anything against him they must speak out now. To which there was usually laughter but no other response.

'One day playing tennis,' he was to relate to us, 'there were five Broeders and myself; we played tennis at the Country Club. And I said, "You know, there's something I don't understand about you chaps. You're all Afrikaners, I'll bet a dollar you're all Broeders. Of course you cannot say if you are or if you're not, but will you tell me something? I've got a lot of English friends and my golly the horrible things I've heard them say about you Afrikaners would surprise you—perhaps it would not! Now please tell me why I have never heard a single Afrikaner at CSIR, including you five, say a nasty thing about the English? Please, it really bothers me, I'd like to know."

'One chap turns to another and says, "Shall we tell him? Sal ons vir hom sê?" And the other says, "Well, I don't think there's any harm."

' "Well, Don, its like this. We feel, you know, that if the Boer War had been won by the Boers, we would still have been a *Bible*-reading nation sitting all over the koppies of the Transvaal, with not another book in the house. Looking after our sheep, shooting game; and we would be reading our *Bibles*. We would never have developed into a nation. The fact that the British won the war and took over the development of this country and then gave us our freedom, made us . . . We knew that the Volk (people) had an opportunity of developing, and we made up our minds to be businessmen—and that's what we've done." '

Craib continued, 'I said, "Look, I know you cannot tell me anything more, I'm not asking questions about the Broeders and so on and so forth. But how is it you still don't say, in spite of all this, you still don't say nasty things about us?" (To which the reply came) . . . "How can we say nasty things about you chaps when you chaps started us on our development? But we did say, one day we would get our country back, but we're not going to get it back by guns, cannons and killing wars, but we are going to get our country back through the vote." Which is what they did.'

Like much of Craib's apparently harmless banter, perhaps there was, beneath it all, a striving for information which would enable him to form a balanced opinion. He was much concerned with relationships between Boer and Briton, as the two components of the white population used to be labelled: although clumsy, Afrikaans- and English-speaking white South Africans would be better terminology. Later, he would use similar methods to help him form his opinions about black-white relationships. Apparently jocular, surely they hid a deeper searching for the truth?

I am indebted to Craib's one-time secretary at CSIR, Mrs EA Shepherd, for much illuminating information on his personality and his scientific influence among research workers. Several years after Don had left the organisation, and in response to her request to interview him on behalf of CSIR, he wrote to her as follows, beginning his letter with a characteristic quip. She was now in a section with the imposing title of 'Publishing, Publicity and Liaison'.

'Hello Evie,

What a terrific—I mean terrific—handle you have to your name these days, and what a pleasant surprise to hear from you. You did say I could call you Evie, didn't you! Or has your new publicity boss put you on your best publicity behaviour?

Now there's one thing about the CSIR—its history can never be complete without an intimate revelation of all your goings on in that august head-quarters building. Compared with *your* goings

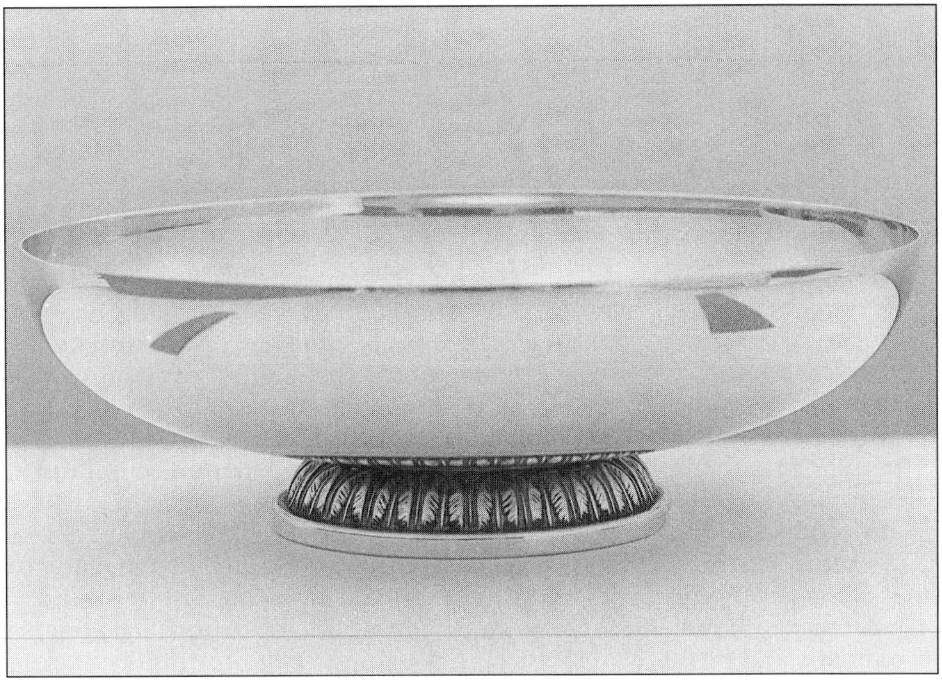

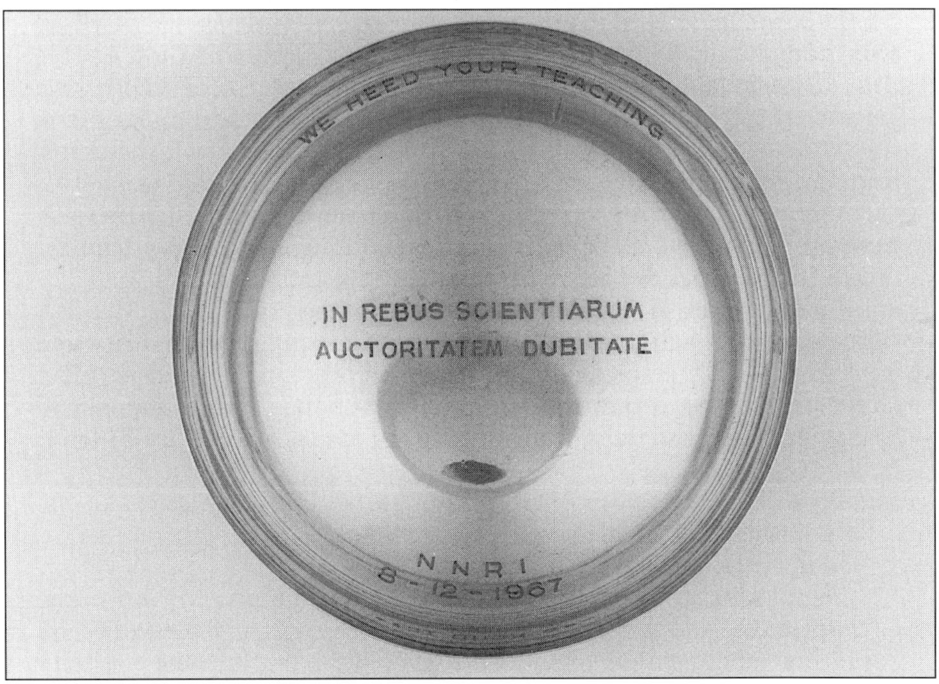

Goblet presented to Craib by the National Nutritional Research Institute on his retirement from CSIR, 1967. It is engraved with his advice to aspiring research workers. (German silver, 10.5×3.5 cm.)

on, you know perfectly well that *mine* amount to nothing at all . . . ' The interview took place at Somerset East.

And a year later, in 1973, he again wrote to Mrs Shepherd with an explanation of the silver goblet presented to him by the National Nutrition Research Institute, an organisation at that time falling under the CSIR.

'One of the jobs I was asked to do at CSIR was to read and to express opinions upon certain papers in preparation for publication, coming from research scientists working at NNRI. In some of these there appeared to be a tendency on the part of the writer to look upon published opinions and statements made by scientists of world acclaim, as though the former, because emanating from the latter, represented fact, truth, or reality, and could not be questioned.

'I objected to this overly respectful attitude on the part of juniors to seniors, or rather to the award of infallibility to so-called "world authorities" by younger scientists on any grounds at all—my standpoint being that in research there are no authorities; experts, yes, administrative authorities yes, but no human authority as to final truth when it comes to explanation of natural phenomena, however recorded.

'After a while there was a measure of agreement between us that when Newton saw an apple fall to the ground he was indeed observing a fact, truth, reality. But when he explained the fall on the basis of what we today refer to as the action of gravity, this gravitational explanation was not, and is not a truth; it is merely a postulate, hypothesis or theory.

'In the end they accepted my little joke that any scientist who accepted as true any explanation of any observed phenomenon without first proving it for himself, was making serious misuse of the funds allotted to him to discover what the truth really was, or is, and should be forthwith removed from his post.

'When the day came to depart, I was deeply touched by the gift of the silver goblet you mention, a delightful present indeed . . .'

Inside the bowl of the goblet presented to Craib by his colleagues at the National Nutrition Research Institute, the inscription (dated 8.12.1967) reads:

'We Heed Your Teaching
In Rebus Scientiarum
Auctoritatem Dubitate'

No better advice could be given to aspiring research workers. He had always doubted authoritative opinion in medicine and did what he could to satisfy himself that there was proof. To stimulate others to heed his teaching was to be his major contribution to medical research in this Indian summer of his life.

Chapter 9

Craib's Jottings and Letter-Writing

Don Craib was a prodigious letter writer. Fortunately he often kept drafts or photocopies of letters he had sent off as well as the replies he received. Craib was also an habitual jotter. Studying both letters and jottings proved a rewarding task for the author since it not only added considerably to other evidence of his intellectual powers but it also revealed aspects of his personality and beliefs which might otherwise have been overlooked. Some of his books and the countless booklets, pamphlets, memoranda and newspaper cuttings which he had kept were sprinkled (usually sparsely, sometimes liberally) with marginal notes and comments.

Elsewhere in this book are quotations from both of these sources. Among his papers, however, was much more that deserves mention; and although these letters and jottings do not contribute to his life's story in a chronological sense, they merit both quotation and comment to broaden the picture of the man. He was meticulous in his choice of language, as shown by the many alterations to drafts of his letters. Sometimes, indeed, there would be several drafts of the same letter. Many of them written to close friends would start or end with some amusing remark or leg-pull. Many of them, too, contained self-derogatory remarks; it is barely credible that he really believed some of them. His warm personality shone through what he wrote. He usually used English, but occasionally he would include a sentence or two in Afrikaans when corresponding with Afrikaans-speaking friends.

Don's letters home from abroad when he was a young man showed his early letter-writing habits. His daughter Mrs Patsy Skinner has early memories of her father's jottings and scribbled note-taking. 'All the years I knew him', she said, 'if a thought came into his head he would write it down, on the back of anything, even his paperback books. You would get the most extraordinary comments made.' Unfortunately, not much material is now available which was written during his active professional life, although he frequently harked back to it in later years. Not surprisingly, his most prodigious letter-writing and margin-jotting period followed retirement from the Council for Scientific and Industrial Research. He was then aged seventy-three, and living at Gardiol, his farm outside Somerset East. All his life he had apparently yearned to live again at his birthplace, but when he moved there for the last time he missed the intellectual stimulus which had flowed from the company of his friends, his medical colleagues and his students. Hence, perhaps, the volume of letter-writing and jotted comments in the intellectually lonely years at Gardiol.

Feeling isolated in this way did not mean that the Craibs lacked visitors. Many and varied were the friends who responded to an invitation or found an excuse to see Don and Doris again at Gardiol, usually to stay with them. Don would certainly make the most of these visits, plying his guests with questions and revelling in the fascinating conversations which stemmed from them. Many of his visitors were fellow South Africans, like Alan Paton, whose more liberal political outlook would ensure lively debate. Some were eminent medical scientists from the United States like Cowles Andrus and George Burch; others, no less distinguished, came from Britain, like Max Rosenheim. All would go away enriched by the experience.

When we visited him there the year before he died, he was mentally alert, his mind almost as clear as a bell. Don's eyesight was failing fast, his brain apparently imperceptibly so. He was as courteous as ever but also as quick-witted and incisive. His twilight had been kind to him. Nevertheless, in weighing up what follows

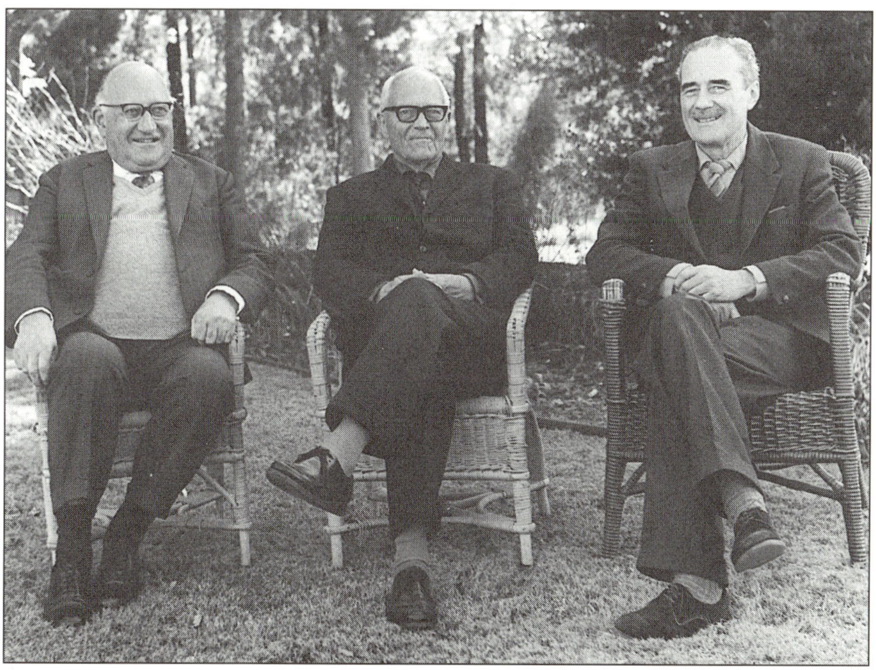

Max Rosenheim, Don Craib and Jack Brock at Gardiol, 1971. (All three had been professors of medicine: Lord Rosenheim at University College Hospital, JH Brock at the University of Cape Town. Lord Rosenheim had also been, for six years, President of the Royal College of Physicians, London.)

the reader must be aware of his age and the possibility that his approach to problems, especially political ones, was more emotional and less detachedly critical than before.

Studying the hundreds of letters found scattered about his study revealed several groups of correspondents. Perhaps first in his priorities were the few survivors among his colleagues at Johns Hopkins, prominent among them being Dr E Cowles Andrus, affectionately named 'Coke'. There were other Americans like Dr George Burch and Dr Raymond Pruitt who became pen friends. Those Americans who were later to see the Craibs at Gardiol usually wrote warmly about their visits to South Africa. Inevitably, South African politics and its complex social problems would then occupy some part of later letters, Don Craib generally stoutly defending what the South African Government was attempting to do. In one of his letters to Craib, Raymond Pruitt perceptively wrote: 'I was delighted with the content of your letter of April 4 (1977). You have very considerable talent for polarizing (and I hope you will not be intolerant of my figurative use of this conventional physical term) the contending elements that relate to any issue of substance. Because you have this capability you are, as I have said before, a masterful *agent provocateur* and a challenge to anyone who indulges in flights of fancy.'

There were many in Britain to whom he wrote over the years. Only a few were from Lewis's research unit. One friend, Sir Bryan Matthews, was with Adrian at Cambridge when Craib and Adrian clashed. Matthews was Assistant Director of Research in Adrian's laboratories at Cambridge at the time of the clash between Craib and Adrian. It would appear from a letter from Matthews to Craib in 1974 that over the years lots of research workers had encountered similar problems with Adrian, for Matthews often had to 'pour oil over troubled waters'. Another colleague with Craib in the Clinical Research Unit at University College Hospital was Dr John Honour, who has been quoted elsewhere. Many of these letters included politics, often concerning Britain's fall from grace (in Craib's eyes) in the 1960s and 1970s over her problems in Rhodesia. Craib was less than generous in his assessment of the rights and wrongs in what is now Zimbabwe, being unequivocally an Ian Smith supporter and failing to acknowledge that there was no simple solution.

The third group were his relatives and other South Africans to whom he would write about a wide variety of subjects. These letters were usually warm and friendly in tone, and, when he did not know the person to whom he was writing, almost always courteous (even when crossing swords with a newspaper editor in the English-language press or a politician who had spoken loosely in his exuberance to get his message across). His letter-writing clearly gave him much pleasure.

In many of these letters a dominant theme is apparent: Craib's passion for exact definition, separating fact from opinion, leading in one way or another to the initial rejection of his research or his personal battles at the University of the Witwatersrand. Craib would deny having been hurt by these several episodes, often writing that 'we had a jolly good laugh about it all'; but the author detected deep-seated hurt, for otherwise surely he would not have relived them so often in his letters. Nevertheless, there was also much fun in his writing.

Don Craib sometimes had long philosophical discussions with his correspondents. It might be said that he was a self-taught philosopher. The professionals would no doubt say that he was very much the amateur. Be that as it may, his thinking in this area is worth looking at.

Over the years, Craib kept up a correspondence with James Schabort, a contemporary of his from Johannesburg who was a consultant gynaecologist. Already aged 85 years, Craib had sent his *Thesis on Truth* for comment. This opened up several other areas of discussion. A letter to Schabort dated 1.9.81 set out Don's views on time and space. His brain, he wrote 'cannot cope with the concept of a future time or a present time' . . . because 'the present time represents a period between future and past . . . and the duration of present time is so infinitesimally brief that it really doesn't exist—for no sooner does time come into existence than it is already past. . . . The future is not only unpredictable for me, it actually doesn't exist in any objective form capable of being perceived via an appropriate sense organ.' Space, he said, 'has no beginning and no end. There is no region in the Universe where space does not exist. There is no such thing as a vacuum if vacuum means a region where there is nothing at all, for it is not possible to get rid of space, and space is an objective something . . . My basic trouble is that I can define nothing that I cannot personally 'perceive' through my sensory system.' Many of Craib's letters included expressions of this sort of thinking. This letter goes on as follows.

> 'I am convinced also that no two humans are, or ever have been, or ever will be identical. I believe that just as a dog's bark or a bird's song is part of the pattern of their bodily behaviour, so also . . . words or language . . . (are) part of every individual's pattern of bodily behaviour. So all I can do in trying to "understand" another person's brain processes is to *infer* from his bodily behaviour and his language just how in my view his brain cells work!
>
> So if someone were to say to me "What sort of chap is James Schabort?", it would never enter my brain to consider any part of your body; may answer would consist solely of what I can recall of your general behaviour and the words you used when I had

> the privilege of your company. In other words, to me you are an abstract inference from what you did to my sensory endorgans and the message they in turn sent to my brain! Inferences that created in me nothing but feelings of respect and affection.'

And then in typical Craibian style, this letter ends with the remark:

> 'You will notice that I avoid using words like personality, spirit, psyche, soul, mind, idea, concept, thought, etc, etc. But that is only because I cannot define them unambiguously!
>
> Yours aye,
>
> Don.'

Craib did not always escape criticism from close friends about his insistence on precise definition of words and phrases. Jock Gear had long worked as his right hand man at the Medical School in Johannesburg and a life-long friendship developed. Jock's clarity of thought and expertise as physician and teacher matched Don's. Unfortunately the bulk of Gear's collected letters were lost after his death. Among the few that are available is a letter in response to a memorandum on academic freedom Craib had sent him in 1972 for comment. 'I go along with your logic and conclusion right to the end . . .', he wrote, 'but, my difficulty is that you have not allowed a licence or 'permissiveness' in the use of words when the word has a meaning somewhat different from its strict derived meaning.' Gear then gives a number of examples, including 'freezing weather', 'second', 'minute', and goes on to tease his one-time teacher with: 'Perhaps you will be amused to be reminded of a lecture you gave to the medical students in the 1930s about 'diabetes mellitus'! If the definition is precisely used, then a patient could have diabetes mellitus in the morning but not in the afternoon!' (Diabetes literally means passing sweet urine.) Jock Gear continued his playful attack by suggesting (tongue in cheek, no doubt) that an opinion poll be set up with large numbers of individuals in many countries, all asked to define 'academic freedom'. Then he jests by asking Craib the question: 'Would not writing and speaking become intolerably longwinded and tiresome if all such words were precisely defined followed by corrected explanations?'

A long letter from Craib to Jock Gear early in 1973 about current controversial issues at Witwatersrand University and others on the wider national scene ends with '. . . it's pleasant to play word games with you—and maybe your friends—in the hopes of getting back daggers of fact and information to stimulate me to battle! The ball is now back to you!' In the same letter, Don had written that a hint is often dropped, when he asked (others) what is meant by 'this phrase or that', not to be so foolish: the phrase is 'perfectly lucid as it stands, there is really no need to question it'. As an example, he added that if he were 'to say that since law and justice have very little in common, the former being nothing more than a very man-made and practical step to protect individual members of organised society from injury at the hands of other members of the same society; whereas the latter is an abstract concept that differs from person to person as to what is right, or fair, or just etc, etc, in some ideal sort of way, differing so widely in fact from person to person that laws supposedly based of so-called justice vary enormously from community to community, and nation to nation or race to race, I am sure to be told that not having studied and practised law, I really know nothing about it and shouldn't display my ignorance by talking about it.' They argued amicably about a variety of subjects besides academic freedom, justice and law; religion and civilisation were included. The stimulus to such pen debates often came from various publications from the university.

Perhaps with his own memoirs in mind, this interchange of ideas and others gave rise to a memorandum Craib wrote in April 1974 which is worth quoting at some length.

'Jock Gear, just retired from a chair of medicine at Wits Medical School, and I have been carrying on a fitful sort of correspondence about Wits for the last year or two. He is about 60 and I am 79. I have always held in highest regard his fearless logic, his honesty of mind, and his patience in dealing with others. He seems to see the heart of a problem and aims his questions well.

'It interests me to know whether at 79 my mind is failing or has failed in its ability to handle, say, a straightforward philosophical problem. So I use Jock as my touchstone or yardstick.

'It is exciting for me to learn from his replies just where I have gone wrong or missed a point; for as long as I can remember I have enjoyed being proved wrong in discussion or argument. It's a good way to learn.

'*Wits Convocation Commentary* comes regularly and I read it with interest. I find I am not infrequently shocked not by what I read, but by the fact that opinions there, and so publicly expressed, seem to be so invalid or unrealistic. This disagreement on my part surely points to serious cerebral deterioration. So I use Jock as my doctor to find out what is going on!

'The technique is to pick on impressive words and phrases published by high ranking Wits intellectuals in senior appointments, and to find fault with them on grounds of ambiguity or sheer semantic carelessness. At times Jock's replies are encouraging; at times not.

'The crunch came a few weeks ago at East London when, referring to a recent letter of mine to him, he threw the ball into my court by saying: "But Don, tell me, why do you concern yourself with Wits affairs of which you do not approve? What do you expect to gain? Do you think you're doing any good?" Or again: "Do you really think any great harm is done when the Dean of Law makes the statement that in a certain case 'justice was done' when perhaps it would have been more accurate, semantically speaking, if he had said 'the requirements of the law were carried out in full'?"

'Of course I saw Jock's point at once. It was a good one. Does it matter what Wits intellectuals say? And who cares anyway?

'The funny thing is that I have been testing myself out against two other yardsticks as well as Jock Gear; one the principal of an English (language) university, the other the ex-principal of an Afrikaans university.

'As the result of Jock's question I now see my dilemma clearly. It flows from the concept of INTEGRITY, and is allied to an uncontrollable, or, in physiological language, conditioned feeling of shame that overcomes me when highrating English-language academics or intellectuals do things or make statements that strike me as unworthy of ancestral characteristics that once filled me with pride.

'Worship of these, as a small boy, made it axiomatic that unless one day one were admitted to Trinity College, Cambridge, one would have to admit oneself a failure!

'It was worship of these that during World War 1, and for no other reason, I performed sufficiently well to earn three decorations for bravery in battle.

'The ancestral characteristics in mind are covered by the word integrity. A word which, not to labour the point, contains something of the essence of the following words: honesty, uprightness, virtue, rectitude, probity, conscientiousness, honour, goodness, principle.

'That one's ancestors indeed possessed these characteristics may well have been nothing more than a dream, the result of schoolboy reading in the Gill College library.

'Nevertheless they still underlie a pattern of behaviour one expects from an English-language university in this country. Shades of Kipling! How certain English-language academics, judging by their public performance, must smile at so endearing a naivety! And that in an academic world seemingly, and without a qualm, jargon (is their) acceptable stock in trade.

'An academic with integrity is surely a person who doesn't wilfully deceive, or consciously equivocate. His purposes are honest and direct; not devious or ambiguous or misleading. If it is pointed out to him that his words or actions constitute doctrine that is not above reproach, he will reflect upon the matter, perhaps be grateful for the tip, and reform if need be.

'But it is precisely here that I have gone astray. I thought that academic integrity mattered. *Convocation Commentary* proves otherwise. Academic integrity implies a war continuously against ambiguity and jargon. There is no sign of that war at Wits . . .'

Rather pompous stuff, no doubt! But it should be remembered that Craib wrote this without leaving evidence of what he intended doing with it. It might be taken as his credo for living. And surely it helps those interested in his life's many controversies to understand why he did what he did. He constantly attacked the use of jargon in speech. It was the subject of his graduation address to the College of Medicine of South Africa when he received an Honorary Fellowship, an occasion when the author delivered the citation.

Don Craib often wrote to Jock's elder brother James Gear, whose friendship was to last almost half a century. After Craib's death, the author discussed him with James Gear, who kindly offered to contribute a memorandum which has been most helpful. Describing Craib's advent to the Medical School, Gear wrote that 'the new professor was young and active and radiated energy, but it soon became apparent that his knowledge of medicine as expounded in the textbooks was more limited than that of his predecessor. He made it clear to his students that, as he himself put it, he was as ignorant as they were and that they had to learn together. He soon inspired his students with his enthusiasm to gain knowledge and soon the library was full of students looking for answers to the question he had asked them. He was an inspiring teacher and in time the students—nearly all of them—almost worshipped him . . . Scepticism was an emotion that he showed towards the generally accepted concepts of disease and he questioned many dogmas and took a mild delight when he had confounded the upholder of a dogmatic opinion. Many recall that he was one of their best and most stimulating teachers.' A number of letters between them are extant. Sometimes their correspondence included political comment but there was little debate since James and Don had a similar political outlook. A quiet, thoughtful man of great ability, James Gear earned considerable kudos at home and abroad for his expertise and published work, mostly microbiological or viral, in the field of tropical medicine.

James Murray, also a pathologist, with a distinguished career at the South African Institute of Medical Research, was another medical colleague on Craib's extensive list of correspondents. Many of Don's memoranda about truth, academic freedom, and the controversies about his own research were discussed, Murray's comments always being fair, to the point, and full of wisdom.

The author's written exchanges with Don Craib usually concerned the problems of the medical school at the University of Natal, but the main themes of Craib's life often entered into his letters. Politics was never discussed. This was surprising since it appeared in so many letters to others. Craib knew the author's liberal stance but never taunted him as he did others with similar views. His letters were frequently amusing and often self-derogatory. One of these ended with the remark that 'you once suggested that I might be described as a sort of philosopher—a blow that still causes my blood pressure to drop every time I recall the words! Philosophers are a type of homo sapiens who may be homo but certainly not sapiens. Indeed I've always pictured myself as the very opposite of "philosopher" and according to my dictionary the opposite of philosopher is ignoramus!—a label I greatly prefer to philosopher!' This light-hearted quip would no doubt have annoyed many who did not know Craib's style, but it contained a grain of substance—for Craib—because he would maintain that philosophers often use terms which they do not, or cannot, define. In yet another of his several scrapbooks, this one dated September 1981, the year before he died, I found a passage he had written about philosophers.

'One reason I dislike philosophers', he wrote, 'is that they lead me up the garden path with language that seems too brilliant for mortal man to follow or understand—yet never does the reader receive any real benefit or help from what the philosophers have so brilliantly to say.

'Take world famous Bertrand Russell for example. I sat listening to his philosophical views for many hours before he offered his definition of TRUTH—which he expressed in the following terms:

'"'. . . Truth is applicable primarily to a form of words, and only derivatively to belief. A form of words is a social phenomenon. Therefore the fundamental form of truth must be social."'

As the first of its several meanings of philosophy, the *Concise Oxford Dictionary* gives 'love of wisdom or knowledge, especially that which deals with ultimate reality, or with the most general causes and principles of things'. The author would therefore stand by his description that Craib was 'a sort of philosopher', his search for truth and 'ultimate reality' surely being the vein which runs through his life's story.

The first page of the 1981 scrapbook includes this revealing comment:

'A common greeting when one meets a friend these days is "Hullo, Don, what do you do with yourself all day?" My reply. "Well, man, I've so much to do these days that there's never enough time to do it in!"'

As his chronicler, the author was left in no doubt about his commitment to thinking and writing, from the volume as well as the calibre of his writing. Letters, memoirs and marginal jottings there were in abundance, even when he was aged 85 years. Among these was a long letter to 'Barry Adams and Tom Bothwell'. Dated 7.10.81, the letter ran to 63 pages! He was now almost blind, so he wrote in a bolder hand than previously; but most pages contained at least 100 words, some many more. He was once again concerned with episodes in his past, especially those relating to his years as Professor of Medicine at Wits. Professor TH Bothwell succeeded Guy Elliott and has earned for himself an enviable international reputation for his researches in iron metabolism; but he is equally distinguished for his clinical acumen, his teaching and his leadership within the medical school. Much of what Craib wrote in this long letter has already been related. It was almost as if Don wanted to make sure his many stances were understood (which they are).

He also let it be known that he considered himself a failure; to which Bothwell replied reminding Craib of the legacy he had left behind and telling him, as others had done, that he was ahead of his time in the 1930s and 1940s with his vision of what the clinical departments at a medical school should be like. Several of the relevant paragraphs from Tom Bothwell's letters to Don Craib in 1981 are worth recording.

In one of them, Bothwell recorded that Craib was in the army when he was a student, so his contacts were few. On the first occasion, he wrote, 'you walked into the hospital lecture theatre, pointed a finger at one of the students and asked him to define death. An hour later the debate was still being vigorously pursued. In fact, when the furore surrounding heart donors broke out twenty five years later I had a feeling of *deja vu*. Much of what was said at that time had been anticipated by your teaching session a quarter of a century earlier . . . Why do I and my contemporaries remember a couple of lectures so vividly? It is because it was the first time that we had been invited to think for ourselves and question authority. It was heady stuff—stimulating and great fun too.'

And in another letter, Bothwell criticises Craib's account in this marathon letter with the words that '(you) barely mentioned the clinical and teaching routines you established and the many positive relationships you formed at Wits, particularly with the student body. It is common cause that any doctor, who was a student during your period of stewardship and is asked to comment on those times, speaks of you in a way quite unlike that reserved for other figures of the time— the anecdotes tumble out and with it (sic) the affection and admiration that you instilled in them. They believe, rightly or wrongly, that you taught them an attitude to Medicine that has remained with them and guided them throughout their professional lives.' What more could any teacher want in old age when reflecting on life's ups and downs?

I have examined all the material available concerning which he made marginal notes or comments. Jottings done in this way must often be on the spur of the moment. They might be purely a means of reminding the jotter to come back to this point in whatever is being read. Sometimes, however, they may be the result of more prolonged thought, and thus reflect the writer's considered opinion. To make much of the many hundreds of Craib's jottings would not only be unwise: it would be manifestly unfair.

Nevertheless, a few examples of Don's marginal comments are quoted because they add to what we know of his expressed beliefs and opinions.

He clearly gave a lot of thought to PB Medawar's *Induction and Intuition in Scientific Thought** because the text of his copy of Sir Peter Medawar's *Jayne Lectures* for 1968 is underlined in many places and freely commented upon. Two examples of Craib's comments follow. Medawar's words 'scientific inference' prompted Craib's handwritten footnote—'What is the difference between scientific inference and non-scientific inference?', followed by another note to the effect that Medawar has answered Craib's question several pages further on. The second example is a scribbled comment to Medawar's words '. . . and the diagnosis will be the right one unless the raw factual information was either erroneous or incomplete'. Craib wrote: 'Factual observation cannot be erroneous unless fact is modified by opinion.'

Earlier on Don Craib had subjected to the same critical scrutiny the published text of JH Hofmeyr's *Christian Principles and Race Problems*, the 1945 Hoernlè Memorial Lecture.** In a number of places Don had scribbled 'nonsense', 'false', or 'not true'. I do not believe these comments were more than his private thoughts so what they refer to will not be dealt with. But Craib's admiration for Hofmeyr on the one hand and his apparent dislike for this distinguished South African on the other certainly merit further comment, throwing, as they do, light on both Craib and Hofmeyr.

His clashes with his distant cousin have already been recorded in connection with Craib's appointment as Professor of Medicine at the University of Witwatersrand. In conversation with the author, Craib would sometimes make what seemed to be snide remarks about 'Hoffie', saying that he would tell the whole story some day. This never came about. But jottings and letters found in his study after his death help us understand some of his criticisms and some of his plaudits.

Before publishing *Wits: The Early Years*, the historian Bruce Murray sent Craib excerpts from the manuscript, presumably for his comments. On a large envelope dated 5.5.81, which enclosed copies of these pages, Don had scribbled what appeared to be a draft reply to Murray. 'After a critical perusal of your article', he wrote, 'and long meditation of racial issues at Wits Medical School some 48 years ago, I must frankly admit that your summary of the atmosphere in which vital decisions were taken is admirable'. Then followed more than fifty lines of comment, ending with: 'The theme of this letter is simply that you admire Hofmeyr too much and let him off too lightly.'

In brief, what he had to say was that 'JH Hofmeyr (Hoffie to me)' was a close personal friend during the years 1912–14 and 'less close but still a friend on pretty intimate terms from 1919 to 1948.'

---

*Medawar PB. *Induction and Intuition in Scientific Thought.* London: Methuen, 1969.

**Jan H Hofmeyr. *Christian Principles and Race Problems.* Hoernlè Memorial Lecture. Johannesburg: 1945, Institute of Race Relations, SA.

After 1930, Craib never saw him 'as a man of Christian principle and trustworthy to the death as I had always assessed him before'. As he moved higher in political life in South Africa, becoming Smuts's right hand man before his untimely death in 1948, Hofmeyr— in Craib's opinion— never allowed principle to interfere with expediency. 'To exaggerate a little', Craib scribbled on, 'Hoffie was more of a disaster than an asset to the University of the Witwatersrand during his days of power, and far less of a power for good in the land than published history has made him out to be. He looked down (on) and distrusted everybody, including Smuts . . . His mighty brain functioned like a modern high powered computer . . .' with little empathy for others, he added, or insight into their weaknesses and sorrows. Don believed he controlled Smuts. These, however, were indeed beliefs. Perhaps Craib could have provided proof, but without his having done so they must remain opinion lacking real substance.

How unlike Craib the scientist these comments are! He overlooked or would not concede the moral stand Hofmeyr often took in the difficult field of politics and race relations in South Africa. Moreover, he made these comments without definite proof of his assertions. Craib could not recognise that there are grey areas in life, especially in party politics, where absolute values cannot be applied. His demand for rigid definition of concepts like freedom, honesty, truth, undoubtedly have intellectual merit, but they are not acceptable to the great majority of people. Craib would have been quick to pick up the difference between fact and opinion about Hofmeyr had they been expressed by others. This was, indeed, one of his blind spots.

Chapter 10

Craib—the Man

Don Craib has surely emerged from this attempt at recording something of his life and times as a clear thinker who was never afraid to challenge accepted dogma; a brilliant, if frustrated research worker; a stimulating teacher of medicine; a successful administrator of medical research; a competent and compassionate physician; a warm friend; an excellent conversationalist; and a self-taught philosopher who spent many hours in his later years probing the world about him, reliving his often controversial past, and writing down his thoughts in memoranda which were never published, and in numerous letters, drafts of which he had the habit of keeping. There is little doubt that Craib had been a conspicuously brave soldier, and after his experiences in the trenches in the First World War, he would say that he feared no man. He would fight tenaciously for a cause he regarded as just, sometimes antagonising authority in doing so; yet he believed in the established order. In old age he was never boring. What is perhaps even more important in the twilight of a long life, he usually centered his conversation on others. He was a delight to meet and to talk to. But in private, in his later years, he appears to have brooded over what he took to be his failures. Being human, he certainly had faults.

His professional life was in medicine, his interests catholic.

In his 1969 scrap-book, Don Craib wrote down what might be taken as his philosophy of life. It reads like a soliloquy. Since Craib would have wanted his chronicler to define this term, I quote from *The Concise Oxford Dictionary*, fifth edition, 1964: 'Talking without or regardless of the presence of hearers', used, the definition continues, especially by a character in a play. Don, however, could have had no play in mind because in this facet of the man, he was a very private person—'I write for myself' it may be remembered was scribbled on the cover of this scrap-book, 'private conversations; a haphazard affair'.

Perhaps he had in mind the young poet who died so tragically in Gallipoli, because there are similarities in what Craib wrote to Rupert Brooke's *The Great Lover*, particularly in the lines:

'These I have loved:
                    White plates and cups, clean-gleaming,
Ringed with blue lines; and feathery, faery dust;
Wet roofs, beneath the lamp-light; the strong crust
Of friendly bread; and many-tasting food;

Rainbows; and the blue bitter smoke of wood . . .
Then, the cool kindliness of sheets, that soon
Smooth away trouble; and the rough male kiss
Of blankets . . .'

Don's piece was in neat handwriting, unlike some of the observations and thoughts he had jotted down elsewhere on countless scraps of paper, old envelopes, newspaper cuttings or as comments on magazine articles, reprints or photocopies he had made covering a diverse range of subjects which interested him. The orderly appearance of this passage suggests that he had, for some time, mulled over what he was going to write. I quote at length but not in full.

'I know not what, whence, whither, who nor why I am . . . But I know what I love and what I hate . . . .

'I love the smell of new-mown hay; the sight of a dry dusty lawn newly washed by rain; a tennis court new rolled and marked, net up, in glorious sunshine; the flight of a well hit golf ball, a gobbled putt; the first daffodils in early spring; digging the fruits of the earth and the smell of new turned earth; the flight of a bird; that happy swing of monkeys in the trees; a jackhanger feeding its young and smacking it with a wing when it continues to squawk for food after five worms in a row; clouds gathering and bringing hope of rain to succour the thirsty; a good sermon empty of insults and implications that Providence is both an imbecile and a sadist; a well written book where semantics are scrupulously in the foreground; a problem well presented and indubitably solved; an erudite and objective turn to conversation and opinion; a recognition of assumption wherever it may exist; cleanliness and tidiness imposed by self-discipline and not by unnecessary and sadistic command . . .'

He goes on in this vein, writing of flowers and trees and several rural mind-pictures; of his wife's dinner-parties at their 'table displaying the Vevers' family heirlooms'; her 'cello playing. But unlike Rupert Brooke, there follows a discourse on his hates:

'But I know what I hate and the first is cruelty of any kind; and the second injustice.

'And yet, to recall my unspeakable youth, what hours of cruelty and injustice to the point of obscenity are to be laid at my feet. The things I did to birds and fish and frogs and harmless innocent animals of all kinds, satisfying some deep subconscious primitive hunting urge that my deeply Christian family accepted without condemnation of any kind . . . I hate the killing of insects by the multibillion to preserve our cereals in growth and storage.

'I hate the torture and killing of animals by each other, the activity that underlies the principle of survival of the fittest. I hate the suffering imposed upon all life by disease.

'I hate the printed and spoken lie by responsible persons in high places. I hate the hysterias of youth based on beliefs that rest upon subjective self-deception without objective basis of any kind.

'I hate a university education that lacks the urge to train the young idealistic mind in the basis of sound deduction . . .

'I loathe any human claim to know the "will of God", for who can speak for God and who can equate his silly little mind with whatever is the equivalent in "God"? . . .

'I resent deeply that the *Bible* adds to my confusion and does not reduce it—and deeply too the fact that the great Christian leaders of the present and the past convince one that the background to their thinking is woolly, sentimental, wishful, inconsistent, and that their likes and actions do not fit their needs and dogmas . . .

'I hate the—to me unjust, unfair—differences bestowed by Providence on living creatures—some weak, some strong, some ugly—plain—beautiful, dull—bright—intelligent—stupid. Not that one expects sameness—but at least one expects balance—to have what it takes: so that the overall "joy in living" for each equates out in the end. I hate the thing that makes masters and servants and human ugliness in all its forms—cruelty, egotism, rudeness, incivility, greed, hypocrisy +++, arrogance +++ . . .

'I loathe above all racial differences in man—as well as the difference between man and man . . . I hate the existence of poverty which threatens the achievements of the believers in decency.'

These loves and hates jotted down by Don Craib were followed by a note on one of his favourite themes: freedom. 'Quote: Man was born free', he wrote. 'No greater rubbish (was) ever said or written and quoted and requoted ad nauseam by the self-appointed spiritual leaders of mankind! What less free, more restricted and imprisoned . . . is (there than) the newly born of mankind. If the newborn babe is free, then certainly freedom has no appeal for me, and cannot have for any sane, balanced and intelligent person.'

To get as complete a picture as possible of the man, it is worth looking at a number of Don Craib's likes and dislikes. His love of nature and his compassion need no underlining: they shine out from the above passages. In the closing pages of this book, his manifest joy in 'an erudite and objective turn to conversation', his 'recognition of assumption wherever it may exist' and his insistence on trying to ensure that words used have precise meanings should need little more by way of comment. Many of his hates recur in his letters and his various unpublished memoranda. They merit closer scrutiny.

Some of his 'hates' are related to religious beliefs and practices. When we interviewed him in Somerset East in 1981—the year before he died—we asked him if he was a Christian. After some thought he replied that he was a student of Jesus. Perhaps we should have pressed him to explain the difference or, indeed, if there were one in his thinking. It will be recalled how disturbed he had been as a boy when told by his elders in a strongly Calvinistic family, many of whom were ministers in the Dutch Reformed Church, that the Jews had crucified Jesus, his searches in the *Bible* having shown him that it was in fact the Roman soldiers who did so. This, he said, lead him in search of truth. He was never confirmed into the Dutch Reformed Church of his Murray and Hofmeyr ancestors. He recalled that 'at about the age of ten my mother once said, 'to know thyself is the beginning of wisdom'—a saying that lay dormant in my mind till the time for confirmation into the DRC had arrived. The struggle to accept what we were "told" was true brought into conflict a genuine enthusiasm to conform with knowledge of the truth of oneself and the realisation that one can't cheat God. Result: no confirmation.' His father's denomination was Presbyterian, which, like the Dutch Reformed Church, must have influenced his religious upbringing; but from our discussions with him in 1981 he then appeared to be closest to the Anglicans, sometimes quoting from the forms of service of the Church of the Province of South Africa, which belongs to the Anglican communion.

Whether or not he spent much time in conventional religious practices or challenging what he read or what religious leaders said or wrote during his busy professional life, is not known to the author. What is clear from his memoirs and his letters, most of them written in his retirement, is that at this stage of his life he had become deeply concerned with religion: perhaps more as a critic than as a practitioner. He would delight in telling of inconsistencies he had found by comparing relevant passages from the many versions of the *Bible* in his possession: thirteen, he told us. One example is the following. On the Cross, Christ is recorded as having turned to one of the thieves being crucified with him, to say, 'This day thou shalt be with me in Paradise'; but the Apostles' Creed states that Christ 'descended into Hell, and on the third day ascended into Heaven'. Precision about time may not have worried the scribes of the day, but Craib found such disparities most disturbing.

'To state that the *Bible* is the word of God,' he wrote in his scrap-book, 'in the sense that God himself dictated, as it were, the original writings on which the *Bible* of today has been drawn up, is untenable. There is no evidence of any such act on the part of God, whatever the opinions of the churches or theologians may be. Opinions are never a source of proof—but they do offer grounds for assumption. The words "of God" are more correctly interpreted as "about God", a view which far more nearly approaches the truth.'

One of Don Craib's strengths as a teacher of medicine and a research worker was his insistence that words used in speech by his students—and others—had precise meaning. He would often seek clarity in language used in discussion or conversation, as illustrated in the chapter on his period as Professor of Medicine at the University of the Witwatersrand.

Craib would also do so with friends and colleagues. An episode which illustrates this characteristic took place at breakfast in a Cape Town hotel some ten years ago, during a medical conference. Craib was in his early eighties. Sitting with two delegates from abroad and being questioned about South African politics, the author was holding forth on the evils of discrimination, when Craib entered the dining-room and asked if he might join the breakfast discussion, promising not to take part, because, he said, he was a very old man. Before long, however, Don could restrain himself no longer and enquired whether the word 'discrimination' implied something wrong or unfair. Forgetting the pitfalls of loose speech when talking in Craib's presence, the author said quite vehemently that it was certainly wrong and manifestly unfair. 'If I discriminate between you three gentlemen,' Craib said, 'is that wrong or unfair?' To which the author—who should have known better, having been his student some thirty years before, and seen much of him since—replied slightly irritated, that he was talking of unfair discrimination. To which Don Craib quipped, 'Ah! If Barry Adams uses the word "discrimination" he means "unfair discrimination"; now I can follow the discussion.' And an Australian cardiologist fell into the same pit a little later and was playfully reprimanded for confusion in his

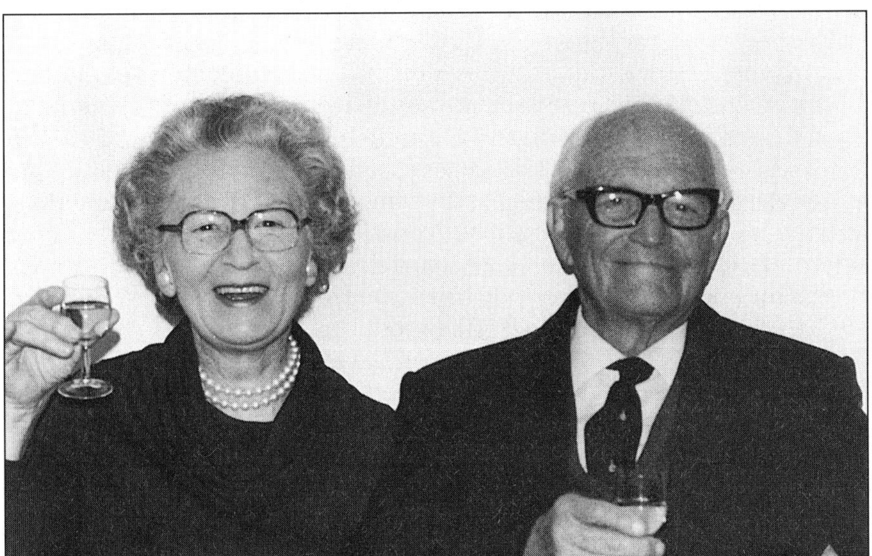

Doris Craib with Don in later years; both in festive mood. Even on occasions like this, Don would mix light-hearted conversation with searching questions.

views of what he meant by the words 'world opinion'. After Craib had left, with conspicuous courtesy as was his custom, the cardiologist added that he now understood what had made Craib the outstanding research worker he must have been to have put forward his doublet hypothesis fifty years earlier.

'All my thinking', Craib wrote, 'seems to be in terms of memory pictures.' When words could be related to facts he had no difficulty in understanding them. For instance, he said, he could understand the word 'sap' and the concept of how it reached the top of a tree by relating it to tiny tunnels or channels up which it ascended. These structures would be made up of cells like those he had seen under the microscope, and they would secrete fluid and push it upwards to a cell barrier, where other cells would again secrete it into yet other channels. Thus he could think about and understand the word 'sap' in terms of memory pictures, and the phenomenon of the ascent of sap in plants could be scientifically explained. But there was a whole series of words which had worried him for much of his life. When he thought about them he had difficulties because he had no memory pictures as a base for his thinking. The words that particularly exercised his mind and were of deep concern because he could not define them as might be expected of a scientist, were words 'such as nothing, zero, infinity, God, time, eternity, heaven, hell, ether, soul, mind, thought, ideas, and a hundred others . . .' And prominent among these was 'freedom'.

Don Craib often pondered the meaning of 'freedom' and held strong views about the concept of the word, particularly in the political sense. There is no greater rubbish, he had written in his 'hates', than the oft-quoted statement that man is born free.

He clearly gave this word and what it means a lot of thought. He could think of no memory picture of anything which was free and therefore unrestricted. The newborn babe is certainly not free. No man, no animal is free in this strict Craibian sense; all are restricted by the laws of nature. And here Don became highly critical of what he labelled as the progressive, liberal political thinkers of the day. When they talked of freedom, he said, they were talking about something non-existent which none the less must be 'aimed at, striven for, and achieved at all costs!'

All men living in communities were restricted by the laws of their society as well as those of nature. If there were no such laws and no constraints imposed by nature, he would no doubt concede that freedom was possible. 'If the freedom worshippers were to preach of reducing our restrictions by increasing or expanding our permissions, and minimising their attendant sanctions, then I'd be on the ball and avid to hear more. The word right', he continued in the same memoir in his 1969 scrapbook, 'which seems to me to indicate only a special permission, granted either by society or by nature, immediately loses its message or intention if prefaced by terms such as divine, sacred, human, or fundamental, when, as is usually the case, these terms are used to exclude the agency of man himself in the permission granted by society, and which is the only real right that any man can have.'

His playfulness never forsook him, even when composing serious passages such as the one just quoted. For he immediately went on with an amusing example which postulated that the Queen had given her gardener the right to use the Bodleian Library whenever he wished to, picturing the vigorous outcry which would follow the first time the gardener went to the Bodleian. 'What a grand to-do there would be in both Houses of Parliament!' And he went on to say that no one but society as a whole or its representative confers rights, and to each right there is inevitably attached a sanction.

It is in relation to his thinking about politics alone that the author has found considerable difficulty. Whether or not I agree with what seems, from his writings, to have been his particular political stance in the South African context is irrelevant. What is relevant is to try to reconcile his various statements and several other facts with the clarity of his thoughts and the consistency of his actions so evident in all other aspects of his life.

Among his 'hates' he put injustice second only to cruelty. He also wrote that he loathed all racial differences in man. Nevertheless, he admired the leader of the National Party of South Africa, Mr JB Vorster, who was Prime Minister and later became State President. On one occasion when the Vorsters were coming to Somerset East, the Craibs were asked if they would have them to stay at Gardiol, to which they agreed. Later a lasting friendship developed between them. After Craib's death, we found Vorster's picture on a wall in his study with several other photographs which must have meant much to him. Among them were an aerial picture of the battleground on the Somme, and Craib being capped as honorary graduate of several South African universities. The friendship is only surprising to the author because Vorster's government, like his party for more than thirty years, was committed to the philosophy of apartheid, with its unswerving policy of incorporating racial differences in much of its legislation, which is manifestly unjust.

Craib was very good indeed to his black employees at Gardiol. He had also been deeply concerned over the plight of black students when they were first admitted to the medical school of the University of the Witwatersrand in the 1940s. He personally funded a bursary there for the best black student graduating at Wits Medical School. Many years later, when the student body rejected the bursary because it was judged to be discriminatory, Craib transferred his donation to the University of Natal, all of whose medical students were black, to be awarded to the student who improved most conspicuously in the subject of medicine during the clinical years.

But he was clearly worried about the political future of South Africa, with its large majority of black people. He accordingly wrote a piece entitled 'The Legend Island', which he never published. He described it as his conundrum in race relations. Since it reflects his thinking on the subject, this lengthy memorandum is worth quoting in part. What remains is summarized.

'Some 300 years ago,' he wrote, 'established populations in Europe suffered from a variety of discomforts—religious, economic, etc. When they became aware of uninhabited continents across the seas, emigration began to take place on an increasing scale. Sailing ships, filled with emigrants set out across the Atlantic in convoys.

'During the voyage of one of these and at the end of a three-day storm, six ships were washed up on the shores of a large deserted island. The survivors came together and found that there were roughly 200 persons from a district in Europe whose people were characterised by strong religious fervour, immense self-discipline, exceptional enthusiasm for higher education and conspicuous industry. Families were restricted to reasonable numbers and the reason for emigration stemmed not from over-population but from dislike of frequent wars. The remainder of the survivors, also some 200 in all, came from a distant part of Europe with a strongly contrasting background, different language, little interest in education, self-permitted freedoms in every direction, a low standard of living, little interest in industry or trade, given freely to alcohol, but also conspicuously dedicated to religion differing widely in its sanctions and creeds.

'After discussion, the leaders of the two groups agreed that the island be divided in two by representatives of one group and that the other group be given the choice. This was done. The island was highly productive. Seed, implements, etc saved from the wrecked vessels, made life increasingly possible and for several generations the settlers throve.

'At the end of a hundred years, life on the two halves of the island provided great contrast. On one side of the dividing mountain range the standard of living, education, housing, industry, low crime rate were impressive and the population density low. On the other side, the population density and crime rate were high, housing poor, education negligible, industry little, poverty conspicuous. Much of the income of the population derived from temporary work across the border.'

In time, he continued, the disparity between the two groups increased conspicuously. Tensions therefore developed 'on the basis that since one half of the island was over-populated and *therefore poverty-stricken*, a portion of the other should be handed over . . . Inter-group bickering increased rapidly and . . . the possibility of war began to be discussed.

'The situation on Legend Island today is extremely serious. The minority industrialised group maintains that there is no ethical reason that can be put forward to hand over any portion of its agreed-upon possessions to the overcrowded, self-indulgent majority, while the majority maintains that on grounds of human dignity, the equality of man, fundamental freedoms and fundamental rights, the minority group must share the island equally with all. They insist on immediate integration, one government set up on the basis of one man, one vote, and unless they obtain their way, war will be declared and they will take what they regard to be their rights by sheer force of numbers.

'What is your solution to the problem?'

It appears from the whole memorandum that Craib had posed this conundrum following discussions he had had with his niece's husband, 'Daantje' Oosthuizen, Professor of Philosophy at Rhodes University, Grahamstown. Preceding the passage set out above is a paragraph attributed to Daantje, probably a condensed or paraphrased form of arguments on South African political problems they had had from time to time, including the question of 'open' universities. In it Professor DSC Oosthuizen makes some personal accusations and follows them by a question that may well have goaded Don into composing the Legend Island story.

'It seems to me that as you have grown older', Oosthuizen is recorded as having said, 'you have become more conservative. Perhaps you now resist any change whatsoever in the running of this country or its universities. You seem to have lost some of the great love you used to have for students. Haven't you become somewhat fascist or dictatorial in your attitude, perhaps even lost faith in the one man one vote form of government for all forms of society? Do you really accept a principle of government that is based upon discrimination between this type of individual and that?'

When he had written it, Craib sent Oosthuizen the Legend Island story for his comments; but the latter had left the country for the United States and Britain and Craib had received no response by the time Oosthuizen died.

Don also posed the problem to many of his friends and acquaintances. Their replies fell into four categories—those who 'quickly and clearly wrote their answers with obvious conviction and an objective approach'; those who angrily or contemptuously refused to answer because the problem was too unreal; those who fell back on the Scriptures and answered that the situation would be resolved if the islanders would obey the will of God; and those who wanted to amend the question and its laid-down conditions and then send an answer. The last three categories of answer were, Craib alleged, motivated by idealism of one kind or another. They all tended 'to an almost obsessional verbosity in discourse on the so-called freedoms, rights and human dignities to which mankind is divinely or fundamentally entitled, whatever these words may mean. They appear to sit on the fence when it comes to an unequivocal definition of right or wrong, good or bad, as though equivocality in such matters is itself virtually a proof of both virtue and wisdom!'

Craib goes on to say that the problem was posed by and for himself. 'It was the culmination of a long struggle to come to terms with myself and in my thinking, about the inner meaning and general application of the "love thy neighbour as thyself" principle', planted in his mind in childhood. His own answer to the Legend Island problem is in category one: unequivocal and unambiguous.

'For me, therefore, the ethical solution is that the disciplined half of the Island population must fight to the death to maintain law and order and decency, or go under. Without law and order and peace, life for the whole of mankind would be reduced to the level of animals where only the fittest survive—a state of affairs intolerable to persons of education and culture to whom the humanities are more important than the bestialities. If justice prevails the disciplined will win the battle. They should thereafter enforce law, order and discipline on their casual, easygoing, overbreeding neighbours, giving help where necessary in an elder brother sort of way. Self and group disciplines must be enforced where necessary by police and army action upon all who do not cultivate the common decencies on their own initiative . . . All overpopulated areas or discontented groups of human beings, large or small, suffer the consequences of their own wilful, avoidable, self-permissive, undisciplined action. The remedy lies not in blaming or accusing or threatening others, but in helping themselves.'

In this memorandum, Craib stoutly maintained that his solution to this 'hypothetical problem was not, most emphatically not, posed against a background of apartheid or separate development in South Africa'. Elsewhere, commenting on Barnett Potter's book *Black Man the Fault*, in which Craib's Legend Island is reproduced as an allegory, Don had scrawled on a photocopy, 'Skin colour never entered my mind.' But the anguish he goes through is the anguish of many fellow South Africans and it is almost impossible to accept Craib's assertion that he was posing a hypothetical situation not motivated by his own worries about the political future of the country in which he spent most of his life, particularly in relation to black/white politics. It explains his friendship with Vorster and his flirtations, as the author believes they might be described, with the policies of the National Party.

His Legend Island conundrum is surely an over-simplification and too clear-cut in its postulate of two groups, one with all the virtues and the other with all the vices. Craib would maintain it was a useful model and this cannot be denied. What is surprising to the author is the manner in which his solution conflicts with his stated hates—cruelty of any kind; injustice; and all racial differences.

This memorandum also adds to the picture of the times in which Craib lived; and it draws attention to Craib's life-long dilemma of rebellion on the one hand and respect for authority on the other. His rebellious nature came to the fore in his childhood over the literal interpretation of the Scriptures; in German South-West Africa in World War 1; in his challenging the accepted beliefs regarding action currents in heart muscle fibres; and in his vigorous disagreements with the hierarchy at the University of the Witwatersrand. His respect for authority, on the other hand, seems to have cut short his challenges to Einthoven, Adrian and Lewis in that he eventually took the path of withdrawal rather than pursuing his conviction that his research was right and theirs wrong; withdrawal from Wits rather than applying again for the Chair of Medicine at Wits when it was converted from a part-time post to a full-time one, although he had always strongly advocated the latter; and perhaps his admiration for authority in the form of Mr Vorster when he could not have been unaware that many of the policies of the government of which Vorster was the head conflicted with his own stated beliefs.

Here, surely, some of Craib's expressed ideas were at odds with others.

Don spent much time in his later years over the concept of academic freedom. This phrase assumed particular importance when the government of the day curbed the right of universities in South Africa to admit whomsoever they wished. The legislation was enshrined by Parliament in the form of *The Extension of University Education Act, 1958*; the terminology used in the title and the contents were most upsetting to the English-language universities, Cape Town, Witwatersrand, Natal and Rhodes. The main object of the Act was to achieve separation of the black races from the whites in university institutions. After various vigorous protests by the opposition in Parliament, and by Senate, Council and academic staff associations in each of these universities, annual Academic Freedom lectures were set up. Speakers were usually distinguished academics or men and women who had achieved national or international prominence.

One of the lecturers was an old friend of Don's, EG Malherbe. Dr Malherbe was renowned as an educationalist. A man of liberal views, with a delightfully frank disposition which endeared him to many, he had distinguished himself as Director of Military Intelligence during the Second World War, having been placed there by General Smuts himself. Malherbe was subsequently a most successful Principal of the University of Natal. His output of articles and published addresses was prolific; and his magnum opus, *Education in South Africa* in two volumes (1925 and 1977) is invaluable in its field. 'EG' or 'Ernie', as he was affectionately known, was also a fearless critic of his fellow-Afrikaners in government whenever he considered their statements or legislation conflicted with what he believed was in the best interest of university education, or pointed to a tightening rather than a loosening of the laws separating the races of the country. He and Don were the same age and were long-standing friends.

Malherbe gave the Academic Freedom lecture at the University of Cape Town in 1973. It is reproduced as an appendix to his book *Never a Dull Moment,* published in 1981. Craib took a photostat copy which he sent to the author. Malherbe's introductory remark that he would 'not try to do what professors usually do, namely, to give a definition to the term under discussion' raised sharp criticism from Craib. These lines were heavily underlined. Don was always scornful of those who would not define what they were talking or writing about. Nevertheless, from surviving letters between these two men, it is clear that each held the other in high regard. Sometimes Craib would taunt Malherbe for his expressed views on politics—and the warm-hearted EG was always outspoken in this regard; but Malherbe would write back that he would not be drawn by his old friend. 'I won't react to all your provocative utterances,' he wrote to Don in 1975, 'either to agree or to disagree. All I can say is that many a practising physician has testified to your effectiveness as a teacher . . . by virtue of this gift of being thought-provoking.'

In 1974 the Academic Freedom Committees of the Universities of Cape Town and the Witwatersrand published a booklet under the title *The Open Universities in South Africa and Academic Freedom.* In Craib's study after his death was found a heavily annotated photostat copy. The committees included such well-known academics as GR Bozzoli, JF Brock, DJ du Plessis, Sir Richard Luyt, Phillip Tobias, David Welsh and Monica Wilson. To Craib, two of their opening sentences must have been like a red rag to a bull: 'The authors of this publication wisely elected not to confine the limits of their concern by an exclusive definition of academic freedom. Instead, they emphasized "the four essential freedoms" of a university, namely, the right of a university "to determine for itself on academic grounds who may teach, what may be taught, how it shall be taught, and who may be admitted to study".' Craib underlined most of this. His annotation reads: Sheer nonsense in engineering, medicine, forestry, etc. He would say, for example, that the South African Medical Council lays down the broad structure of the medical curriculum and provides guidelines; not the universities. And so his relentless criticism continues. 'What is a free society?', he would scribble across a page; 'What are the rights of a university?' on another; and so on. Most readers of the booklet would be left in no doubt, in general terms, what this committee was advocating. But for Craib, such generalisations would be unacceptable. He would demand precision in speech and writing: a highly desirable goal, no doubt; but language is not capable of precise definition of every word employed. The *Shorter Oxford English Dictionary* gives eleven definitions of the word 'freedom'. Normal accepted licence would surely allow the writer or speaker to choose any one of these to suit his intended meaning. 'Exemption from arbitrary control; independence; civil liberty', this dictionary's second definition, would suit the purposes of the authors of *The Open Universities in South Africa and Academic Freedom* very well; but not Craib. Perhaps this is why he published so little although in private he wrote much.

Craib would have challenged the author in his use of the words 'manifestly unjust' above (in the discussion of Craib's 'hates' and his friendship with Vorster), just as he challenged, by his scribbled comments, the committee of *The Open Universities in South Africa and Academic Freedom* wherever they used terms such as 'academic liberty', 'rights', and 'academic and human freedom are indivisible'. He had received an honorary degree from the University of Natal so was sent invitations to its most important functions. The annual Academic Freedom lecture was one of these. One year he wrote to the Principal, Professor Francis Stock, suggesting a public debate between himself and the Professor of Law on the meaning of the words 'academic freedom': a challenge which Stock prudently declined to accept on behalf of his university!

Craib's apparent obsession about the meaning of words may readily suggest a tedious nature; but friends and acquaintances never found him so. There was always humour mixed with challenge.

The theme running through much of his life's story is Don Craib in search of truth. In his youth he recalled that he was very worried about truth and left school with the belief that truth is in no way different from fact, reality, event. 'As soon as a person made a statement', he had told us, 'that did not agree with or was not consistent with fact, reality, event, it was not truth'. In a busy career involving electrophysiological research, teaching and practising clinical medicine, and research administration, Craib stuck to the facts. Particularly in teaching medical students, he would insist on a clear separation of fact from opinion. It was only fact, reality, event that equated to truth. Writing about medical students when he was Professor of Medicine at the University of Witwatersrand, he said that 'for three years we were students together in search of truth about man, his mind and his body. If bluff there was, then bluff had to be called without respect of persons.' Some of his colleagues would certainly be ruffled. Searching for the truth about action currents in cardiac and skeletal muscle eventually led to clashes with Sir Thomas Lewis and abandoning his first love, research, rather than compromising his principles; and the break with Lewis, whom he admired as none other, must have been a major crisis in his life. Truth, he jotted down many times in his various scrap-books, does not depend on the mind of man. It would exist in the universe without the existence of man.

What is perhaps most significant is the frequency with which his search for the meaning of truth appears in his voluminous papers.

At the age of eighty he was still writing to a wide range of friends, former colleagues and even less well-known acquaintances, posing the question: 'Would you please give me one instance of truth which is not at the same time a fact, reality, event.'

Most of those who received this letter did not reply. The few who did admitted failure. One or two replies were amusing but the question was almost always evaded in one way or another.

A former Professor of International Relations at the London School of Economics wrote: 'I'm glad, Don, your question this time was so easy. You see truth is like goodness and beauty. No one can define these words, but everybody knows exactly what they mean.'

A senior intelligence officer on Montgomery's staff during the Second World War answered that 'it is not possible to define truth as though truth stood for something concrete. You see every person on earth has his own idea of the truth!'

Oliver Schreiner, at one time Chief Justice in South Africa, and a good friend of Don's, was asked the same question. 'All your life as a judge,' Craib had quipped in a letter to him, 'you have had people before you swearing to tell the truth, the whole truth, and nothing but the truth. Please tell me what you mean by the truth?' To which Chief Justice Schreiner replied that he was sorry, he could not give a cast-iron definition.

Sir Richard Luyt, at the time Principal and Vice-Chancellor of the University of Cape Town, when challenged what he meant by truth in speeches he had made in Israel, replied that he used the word truth 'in the sense of knowledge which cannot be faulted, i.e. which responds favourably to all endeavours to establish its accuracy, and which, when tested, cannot be shown to be false'. In a postscript Luyt added a sentence that must have pleased Craib. 'I am sure the American Declaration of Independence is open to the strongest criticism in declaring 'We hold these truths to be self evident—that all men are created equal; that they are endowed by their Creator with certain unalienable rights; that among these are life, liberty and the pursuit of happiness.'

These replies must have given this questioning man immense pleasure. His pursuit of truth never ended. From it he derived his manifest enjoyment of life.

Chapter 11

Vindication

Perhaps most people of Don Craib's intellectual calibre, in old age, look back with some regrets on what might have been. Perhaps, too, Don was an unfulfilled genius who had deeper regrets than most about what he would call his failures. He must have written to his sister Ismay about this on his retirement from CSIR in 1968, because Lady Schonland's reply included a very poignant passage which reads:

> 'Your own life has been so noble and so full that it stands entirely justified in its own right. So do not regret your decisions in the past. You would of course have been a very great figure in the medical research world if you had stayed in research. But you were a very great figure anyway and have at any rate served South Africa very well—with the training of medicals, the organisation of research, and the actual patients to whom you gave life and courage.'

Praise indeed when it is remembered that Ismay and he had crossed swords many times in the past, particularly over their political beliefs, which were poles apart. As he got older Don's views became more right wing, as we have seen; hers were more liberal, unacceptably so to him.

It is surprising that he continued to hark back in his twilight years to what he interpreted as his scientific rejection in the 1920s and 1930s by Einthoven, Adrian, Lewis and others—the 'Nobel prizewinners' he would call them, or the 'men who held the money bags', for his cardiological research eventually received wide acceptance and much praise.

First indications that opinion had changed about the validity of his research on action currents emanating from isolated cardiac muscle came to him in 1947. A Mexican cardiologist, Dr Demetrio Sodi-Pallares had sent him a book which included 'the first evidence ever to reach me that my researches of some 20 years before had ever been considered seriously by any living person'. This is how Craib expressed it in a later letter to Pallares. In another book, *Deductive and Polyparametric Electrocardiography*, published in 1970, Pallares wrote:

> 'It was during those evolutionary years that I became acquainted with the "Doublet Theory" of WH Craib. His work made a profound impression on me. I have always maintained that some

minds are prone to be guided by divine inspiration and that young man, in his intense search, came to understand the activation process of the heart as no one else before.

'His unyielding sustenance of the truth generated a determined opposition of certain reigning interests, putting an end to the scientific career of this brilliant scientist, named WH Craib.

'Not having known Dr Craib personally has been a regret in all my life. I extend to him my greatest admiration. Although I did not have the privilege of knowing him, time and distance have acquainted me to a point where I am sure he is a marvellous person who deserves respect and deference from all scientists. I trust these lines dedicated to him, that carry the high regard that I hold for him may help restore his faith in scientists once again and also hope that he will forgive those who betrayed his talented scientific knowledge.'

A few years later, Don Craib should have been even more reassured when he received a copy of a paper on 'Doublets, Dipoles and the Negativity Hypothesis' by Raymond Pruitt* containing much praise for Craib's work. Pruitt writes that he first became aware of Craib's existence when he joined Frank Wilson's laboratory in 1946 to study ventricular excitation and injury and was told at the outset to read Craib's articles. Pruitt had inscribed his paper 'To William H Craib, with esteem and affection. Your understanding and support made this paper possible.' Its full title described the paper as 'An historical note on WH Craib and his relationship with FN Wilson and Thomas Lewis.' Several passages are quoted here, Pruitt's words expressing clearly and succinctly the very considerable impact of Craib's researches. Referring to Robert Browning's comments about 'a small event' in 'Pippa Passes', Pruitt introduced his subject with the words:

'Viewed within the macrocosm of science's history, the doublet-dipole theory of Craib and Wilson was 'a small event'. But within the microcosm of the evolving science of electrocardiography it was a revolution. That theory, when combined with knowledge of ventricular excitation as propounded by Lewis, permitted the investigator and the clinician to introduce logic into interpretation of the ventricular electrocardiogram. . . .'

Pruitt went on to outline Craib's story, and analysed the relationship and the contributions of Craib, Wilson and Lewis. He summed up with a passage which reads as follows:

'If these comments are laudatory of William H Craib, then they are as they should be. His substantial contributions to our

*Pruitt, RD. *Johns Hopkins Med J*, 1976: **138;** 279–288.

understanding of the ventricular electrocardiogram seem not to have been accorded their deserved place in the history of this science . . .

'. . . I would not pretend to measure the performance of Lewis, Craib, and Wilson, either in isolation or in relationship each to the other. By their several and distinctive efforts, they contributed to our understanding of ventricular excitation, of doublets, and of dipoles. Perhaps this new manner of speaking they initiated altered little the perceptions and conclusions of physiologists generally; but to the clinical cardiologist, that novel electrocardiographic dialect became the language of reason which led on to understanding, discovery, logic, and, *mirabile dictu*, computerized interpretation.

'A small event? Yes, only a small event, but within the confines of its application it encompassed the substance of revolution and a portent of order and beauty.'

The same year (1976), Don accepted an invitation to attend the 7th European Congress of Cardiology in Amsterdam, where he was to be honoured. Vindication had now come in full measure. The President of the congress, Professor D Durrer, who had first written about Craib's doublet in 1952, made the award.

'At last I have found you,' he said, 'after hunting high and low for nearly 30 years! I first became a fervent admirer of yours at a time when I had little mathematics and less physics and was trying to learn something of the mystery of ventricular depolarization. Your article in 1927 in *Heart*, and your Medical Research Council monograph of 1930 gave me clear cut answers to some of the problems I faced in those days. You opened my eyes wide with your analysis, and the study of your work was a revelation . . . Your work caused a revolution in electrocardiography and was a turning point which initiated a scientifically sound approach to this important field of cardiology . . .

'You heard your work qualified as an egregious failure. But times have changed: everyone familiar with the fundamentals of electrocardiography recognises the importance of your work and does so with deep gratitude.

'It is my privilege to express the feelings of European cardiologists but they are also those of cardiologists all over the world.'

Leo Schamroth was a graduate of the University of the Witwatersrand after Craib's time but fell under his influence. He was Professor of Medicine at Baragwanath Hospital and became an international figure in the field of electrocardiography. Like Craib, his forte was clarity of thought and expression. Despite his early death in 1988 after two major illnesses, which he bore with conspicuous fortitude, his obituary notice in *The Lancet* credited him with 18 books and monographs and over 300 scientific publications. The mind boggles at the ability of any man to be so prolific in his writing, especially in the critical field of medicine. One of his books, *Introduction to Electrocardiography*, written and illustrated with great clarity, as was his habit, had the distinction, the obituary tells us, of 'being the book most often stolen from medical libraries throughout the world!' He qualifies in good measure to be included in the life and times of Don Craib for two reasons. The one is that, having similar intellectual qualities and medical interests, he and Craib became close friends. Many letters passed between them. The other reason is that this distinguished South African cardiologist took up the cudgels about the initial rejection of the doublet hypothesis.

In the late 1960s he began writing about Craib's contribution to electrocardiography and in the mid-1970s began giving a most amusing public lecture with the title 'The Trial of William Craib'. It was no doubt inspired by Schamroth's reading of Craib's private document *In Defence of Honour* which Craib had submitted to the Rockefeller Foundation. A dozen or so copies were also circulated to friends, the author included. Both took the form of imaginary court scenes. Like Craib's, Schamroth's aim was vindication. Most of its substance has been dealt with in the pages of this account of Don Craib's life and times. The highlights need no further emphasis. One point emerges about which Schamroth made rather much. This was Craib's perceived allegation that he had been accused of plagiarism, that a decade or more before Craib's research was carried out and published, Einthoven had proposed such a theory; and furthermore, that Frank Wilson was given the sole credit when he published his work on the dipole in 1933. None of the allegations stands up to critical scrutiny and Craib certainly bore no resentment towards Wilson. The author could not put it better than Howard Burchell did when he wrote: 'I think the matter should rest with praise (*in excelsis*) for both Wilson and Craib.'

Two other points made by Schamroth are worth including. He summarised Craib's research as having demonstrated that 'the activation front of the heart had a positive head and a negative tail, and this activation front with a positive head and a negative tail Craib termed the doublet or the dipole', adding that Craib preferred the term doublet. The second point Schamroth made was his opinion about the impact of the doublet hypothesis: '. . . not only did it dominate electrophysiological thought thereafter, but it enabled the rational, deductive and logical interpretation of the electrocardiogram.'

Elsewhere in the world of scientific medicine, others joined in the acclamation accorded Don Craib by Durrer, Pruitt and Schamroth. An exhaustive list would be tedious but some should be recorded here. Perhaps most valued of all was his election in 1977 to the Johns Hopkins Society of Scholars. The citation at the Commemoration Day ceremony when the honour was bestowed included the statement that 'it was during his years in Baltimore and London that Dr Craib made exciting discoveries about the fundamental origins of electrical signals in the human heart, and from these developed his original work on the electrocardiogram. At first there was outright opposition to his theories, but he persistently maintained the validity of his experiments and his views ultimately prevailed.' It is also worth adding that before the congress in Amsterdam, three South African universities, Cape Town, Witwatersrand and Natal, recognised this outstanding man by conferring honorary doctorates on him, and the College of Medicine made him an Honorary Fellow. Later, the Universities of Stellenbosch, Port Elizabeth and Rhodes followed suit. There were other honours. The South African honorary degrees must have meant much to Don, for photographs of some of the ceremonies adorned his study walls, and there too was the impressive aerial picture of the western front in 1916 at the time of the battle of the Somme. The various episodes so reflected were clearly deep emotional events for Craib, as was the presence on his bookshelves of Lewis's *The Mechanism and Graphic Registration of the Heart Beat*, which he would take out and show his medical visitors when talking of his rewarding but turbulent years with that great scientist.

Craib's admiration for Lewis was clearly undimmed by the events at University College Hospital fifty years before; but he never appeared to forgive the hurt he attributed to Adrian and Einthoven, both Nobel prizewinners, and HB Williams, a leading American cardiologist of the day. Before the Atlantic City meeting in 1926, Williams is said to have told EP Carter (Craib's sponsor) that 'if Craib's work went on, it would put the Hopkins laboratory in disgrace'.

What Don never really came to terms with was the reality about scientific revolutions and the time scale of their acceptance. As TS Kuhn has put it, new theories regularly evoke resistance from some of those authorities upon whose fields they impinge—in Craib's case, Lewis, Adrian and Einthoven. For them, the new theory 'implies a change in the rules governing the prior practice of normal science' and inevitably reflects on much of their own work already published. New theories are seldom mere increments of existing knowledge. Their assimilation means 'the reconstruction of prior theory and the re-evaluation of prior fact', a revolutionary process which needs time and is frequently too slow for the inventor. Lewis, Craib recalled, told him that his work was 'undermining the house' he had so painstakingly built and recorded in his great book *The Mechanism and Graphic Registration of the Heart Beat*; and so working together became no longer possible.

'Whatever happened to William Craib?', the young Raymond Pruitt asked his mentor, Frank Wilson, when he had read Craib's articles and heard the story up to the time Don left Lewis's research unit. Craib was, of course, lost to electrophysiological research, in which field he might have continued to make outstanding contributions, given his original mind and his clarity of expression. This book tries to answer Pruitt's question about his subsequent career, and to evaluate his experiences and his philosophy of life in the times in which he lived. His life was never dull, his influence on others immeasurable.

Index